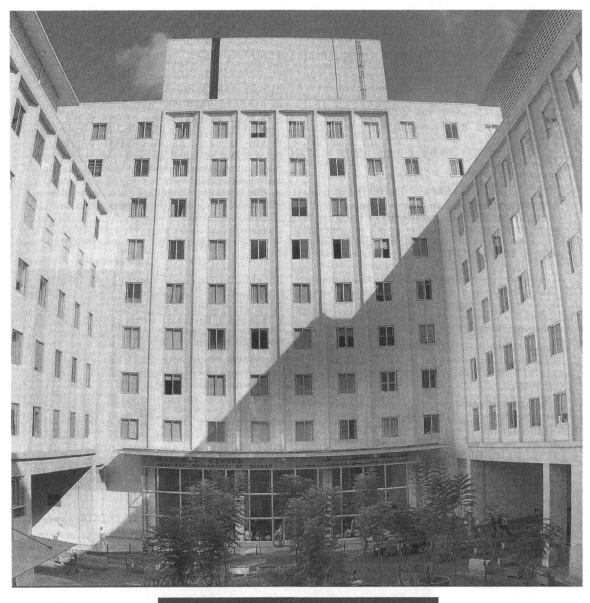

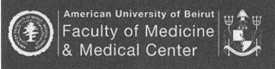

Photo credit: AUBMCNEWS Summer 2008 2003 Vol. 12 No. 3 p. 22

CLINICAL MEDICINE RESEARCH HISTORY at the AMERICAN UNIVERSITY of BEIRUT, FACULTY of MEDICINE 1920-1974

Mounir(Munir) E Nassar, M.D., FACP

WESTBOW
PRESS
A DIVISION OF THOMAS NELSON
& ZONDERVAN

WestBow Press books may be ordered through booksellers or by contacting:

WestBow Press
A Division of Thomas Nelson & Zondervan
1663 Liberty Drive
Bloomington, IN 47403
www.westbowpress.com
1 (866) 928-1240

Because of the dynamic nature of the Internet, any web addresses or links contained in this book may have changed since publication and may no longer be valid. The views expressed in this work are solely those of the author and do not necessarily reflect the views of the publisher, and the publisher hereby disclaims any responsibility for them.

Any people depicted in stock imagery provided by Thinkstock are models, and such images are being used for illustrative purposes only.
Certain stock imagery © Thinkstock.

ISBN: 978-1-4908-3279-1 (sc)
ISBN: 978-1-4908-3278-4 (e)

Library of Congress Control Number: 2014906088

Printed in the United States of America.

WestBow Press rev. date: 5/6/2014

For those physicians past and present whose historical pioneering discoveries improved the health of all of humankind.

To the physicians of the Faculty of Medicine at the American University of Beirut who made research history in the making of the golden age of the University Medical Center, vibrant and well, from 1920 to 1970. In particular, Dr. Sami I. Haddad, Dr. George Khayat, Dr. Stanley Kerr, Dr. George Fawaz, Dr. Henry Badeer, Dr. Hrant Chaglassian, Dr. Philip Sahyoun, and many others listed with their published papers in this manuscript.

Also, to notable American physicians—in particular, Dr. Joseph J. McDonald, Dr. John L. Wilson, Dr. Virgil Scott, Dr. Calvin Plimpton, and Dr. Samuel Asper.

To Dr. Arthur Selzer and colleagues (San Francisco) for making it possible to undertake my American Heart fellowship program in clinical cardiology.

To Dr. Eugene Braunwald (Harvard) for his important numerous contributions to cardiovascular pathophysiology and his clinical contributions to the practice of cardiovascular medicine.

To Alfred E. Nassar, BA 1952, MA candidate, Faculty of Arts and Sciences, AUB, Economics Department; formerly associate director in the administration's Business Computer Division of AUB.

At Columbia University College of Physicians and Surgeons, New York, New York, to Dr. Hamilton Southworth, Dr. Dickinson W. Richards (my mentor), Dr. Andre Cournand, Dr. Richard Stock, and Dr. Robert B. Case. Also, to Dr. O. Robert Levine and Dr. Robert B. Mellins, at the Cardiorespiratory Laboratory, who, under the leadership of Dr. A. P. Fishman, were pioneers of basic scientific research with the work they accomplished measuring the water space of the lung.

To the Faculty of Medicine-Surgery at the Methodist Hospital, the teaching hospital of Baylor University College of Medicine in Houston, Texas, as it was known then, with its leader, Dr. Michael E. DeBakey, the noted pioneer cardiovascular surgeon in open-heart surgery and aortic aneurysms, who led the way for the inception of the first modern surgical intensive care unit.

With gratitude to Dr. Ingmar Cullhed of the Akademiska University Hospital at Uppsala, Sweden.

I owe a debt of gratitude to all of those physicians, past and present, whose individual contributions to teaching and clinical research made a lasting impact on the history of medicine and its research, including my medical education. I believe it is only meritorious to include all those physicians who have made my clinical practice and approach to research so enjoyable.

Finally, in loving memory of my parents, especially my dad, Emile (student, dean of insurance, and lecturer at the School of Arts and Sciences of AUB, and nominated for an honorary BA degree), and my uncle Fuad (BC, 1910), for their patience, encouragement, and support.

Contents

Chapter 4

I would like to acknowledge my indebtedness to Dr. Farid S. Haddad for his love of medical history and his invaluable published contributions. Without his encouragement, this book would not have been written.

I would like to thank my brother, Alfred E. Nassar, for his help at a time when the use of computers was in its budding stage, and for reviewing the statistical analysis of lung function norm formulas of Lebanese children.

My gratitude goes to Kenneth Sympson for his technical advice.

Thanks to Aida Farha, librarian specialist at the Saab Medical Library, the Faculty of Medicine of the American University of Beirut (AUB), for her expert help in making available research sources.

As a graduate of International College and of both the Faculty of Arts and Sciences and the Faculty of Medicine of the American University of Beirut (Beirut, Lebanon), I have been impressed by the quality and high caliber of the education that I received. I believe that all AUB graduates, regardless of what discipline they pursued, share my opinion.

I am very proud to have received my education and higher professional education at the American University of Beirut and its Faculty of Medicine, and to have been in a small way engaged in its scientific preclinical and clinical research that have prompted me to write this book documenting their origin and progress.

I was intrigued that research was a realized development to have taken place among recognized publications catalogued in the US Medical Congressional Library and the Saab Medical Library of the Faculty of Medicine.

The purpose of this manuscript is to document the early beginnings of medical research from 1920 and its progress until 1970 through what I would like to call the golden age of preclinical and clinical research. My intention is to show that over the years, while medical education was being tuned to a fine level of excellence, clinical research did not lag behind but kept pace with the medical educational curricula.

Chapter 1 contains definitions of types of research—mainly medical research. Also, it has a historical synopsis of the founding of the Syrian Protestant College (SPC). Its forerunner, the Academy Missionary School at Abeih, Lebanon, was established in 1843, headed by Dr. C.Van Dyck. SPC began its educational role officially on December 3, 1866, for higher learning, to graduate local people of the region and other people from all walks of life. In 1868 the medical department was established with its faculty of doctors. The present American University of Beirut campus land was bought as early as 1870, and its acreage acquisition was completed 29 years later with definite walled borders. Between the years 1870 and 1873, College Hall, Ada Dodge Hall, and the medical building were built each for their respective faculty. The medical building became known as C. Van Dyck Medical Building. In 1920, the Syrian Protestant College became the American University of Beirut, in Beirut, Lebanon. My discussion of medical research starts after 1920, though with a few exceptions of earlier work during the period 1866–1929.

Chapters 2 and 3 are a record of the clinical publications of each department comprising the Faculty of Medicine. As much as is possible, I have attempted to comment on certain research papers and their relationship to more recent medical developments.

The clinical research was founded on a rich heritage of the evolving Arab medicine from early times, mixed with American and European clinical research filtering through to the Middle Eastern–enriched clinical research at the university. While a medical resident in 1960, I took up a project of publishing articles of the medical faculty in the first issue of the journal, *The Medical Bulletin of the Faculty of Medicine of AUB.*

I must make the reader aware that in a rich medical environment, scientific and clinical ideas become available for the taking to implement research. It is an excellent modality for medical progress. Such ideas are usually generated in medical rounds on patients, or over lectures, or scouring medical journals for answers to unsolved problems.

Though my book will expand on certain medical research papers (preclinical and clinical research) and their significance, my emphasis will be mostly on clinical cardiovascular research that I was involved with, and with notations on their application to clinical cardiology, in chapters 3 and 4 respectively.

Chapter 4 relates my own journey into medical research starting with a term paper while a junior student. Though not of a medical subject, it launched my interest to become involved in medical research—primarily cardiology.

Mounir (Munir) E. Nassar, MD, FACP

Definitions of Medical Research and Development of the Department of Medicine of the Syrian Protestant College (1868) to the American University of Beirut Faculty of Medicine[1]

Medical research is a diligent inquiry and examination into the discovery and interpretation of data or new knowledge arrived at by experimentation. It is a search for answers to unsolved medical problems.

- There is basic scientific research in medicine, as noted above.
- There are other types of research, such as analysis of collected clinical data or reporting on unusual clinical findings. This is clinical research and/or epidemiologic research, which influences new therapies or preventive measures. Pharmaceutical research includes the search for new chemicals and/or new medications.
- Yet another type of medical research is found in the history of medicine. It is based on old manuscripts and considers documentation of how first medical discoveries were made.

If a man will begin with certainties, he shall end in doubts, but if he will be content to begin with doubts, he will end in certainties.[2]   —Francis Bacon

Knowledge does not advance by verification of true doctrines but by refuting them.[3]   —A.V. Pollack and M. Evans

The truth in medicine is to be likened to Beethoven's unfinished tenth symphony.   —Mounir E. Nassar

The purpose of this paper is to portray, in documentary fashion, how, from the history of the foundation of the Syrian Protestant College (SPC) Medical Department in1868, which in 1920 became known as the American University of Beirut (AUB), basic preclinical medical research

---

1   Stephen B. L. Penrose Jr., *That They May Have Life. The Story of the American University of Beirut 1866–1941* (Beirut, Lebanon: American University of Beirut, 1970); Carlton S. Coon Jr., ed., *Daniel Bliss and the Founding of the American University of Beirut* (Washington DC: The Middle East Institute); John M. Munro, *A Mutual Concern. The Story of the American University of Beirut* (Delmar, NY: Caravan Books, 1977).

2   F. Bacon, quoted in *Oxford Dictionary of Quotations*, 3rd ed. (Oxford, 1980).

3   A. V. Pollack and M. Evans, *JRSM* (1985): 937–940.

and clinical investigative papers became integrated with the primary educational role of the university. Such academic activity occurred at the School of Medicine and Hospital, later known as the Faculty of Medicine and the AUB Medical Center Hospital.

Against all odds, research became established slowly but surely. This is an interesting journey, and one has to begin with an historical narrative to show that medical research at the AUB became an important and integral part of the school's high standards in medical education.

The SPC was founded by Presbyterian missionaries. Foremost among them were Mr. Willis Thomson and, later, Daniel Bliss, doctor of divinity and of letters, who, under the charter laws of the state of New York, opened the doors of the college on a beautiful campus overlooking and extending to the coast of the Mediterranean Sea. The vision of its founder, President Bliss, and the faculty assisting him can be summarized by his own words of December 7, 1871.

> This College is for all conditions and classes of men without regard to color, nationality, race, or religion. A man white, black, or yellow, Christian, Jew, Mohammedan, or heathen, may enter and enjoy all of the advantages of this institution for three, four, or eight years, and go out believing in one God, in many Gods, or no God. But it will be impossible for anyone to continue with us long without knowing what we believe to be the truth and our reasons for that belief.

The motto of the university, inscribed on a marble plaque at its main entrance on Bliss Street, became equally famous: "That they may have life and have it more abundantly" (reference to John 10:10).

Daniel Bliss was born on August 17, 1823, in Vermont and died in Beirut in 1916. He was a devoutly religious man and a missionary-activist by nature. Bliss graduated at the top of his class from Amherst College and Andover Theological Seminary (1852 and 1855, respectively). In 1862, the Board of Commissioners Managers recommended his appointment to the presidency of the SPC. It was officially accomplished in 1866, when the college began its educational functions.

The Board of Commissioners Managers' functions were later taken over by an independent board of trustees, which was incorporated under charter by the state of New York. Its board included the following:

- William A. Booth
- William E. Dodge
- David Hoadley
- Simon B. Chittenden

- ⅄ Abner Kingman
- ⅄ Joseph S. Ropes

At the time, the college faculty concentrated much of its effort on translating the Bible into Arabic. That was started by Ely Smith, Butrus Bustani, Sheikh Nassif El Yazigi, and Yousef Al Asir. It was completed by the latter three scholars, with the help of Dr. Bliss and Dr. Cornelius Van Dyck, who was appointed as the head of the medical department (school) in 1866.

The faculty at that time were the following:

- ⅄ Dr. Cornelius Van Dyck
- ⅄ Dr. George E. Post
- ⅄ Dr. John Wortabet
- ⅄ Dr. Harvey Porter
- ⅄ Dr. Edwin R. Lewis

These courses were taught at the SPC:

- ⅄ Arabic, English, French, Turkish
- ⅄ physical science, chemistry, mathematics, Bible study

The following courses were taught in the medical department:

- ⅄ anatomy and physiology
- ⅄ *materia medica*
- ⅄ surgery
- ⅄ practical and clinical medicine

For several years, courses were taught in Arabic. It was an arduous task for American professors to translate the textbooks from English to Arabic. When the curriculum was changed to English, it was quite a relief to the faculty.

In 1871, with five professors, the department of medicine graduated six medical doctors:

- ⅄ Salim Diab
- ⅄ Salim Furayj
- ⅄ Yusuf Hajjar
- ⅄ Nasir Hatem
- ⅄ Rashid Shukralla
- ⅄ Shibli Shumayyil

What a proud moment it must have been for Dr. Daniel Bliss and the medical faculty of the SPC to grant the diplomas to the graduates. After all, they worked with an operating budget of only $100,000 for the college.

Prior to graduation, the doctors had to submit to an Ottoman medical exam, given by the High Ottoman Port. It must be noted at the outset that the purpose of the SPC—and later the AUB— was to achieve excellence in educating men and women of the Middle East, be it in medicine, liberal arts, or sciences. Conducting medical research was a good second in importance.

After many years of labor and hardships, the buildings were built on a beautiful seventy-two acres in Ras Beirut. The medical environment in the Arab world provided a rich heritage of clinical case histories, which directly or indirectly influenced the physicians of the Faculty of Medicine of the AUB to launch their own clinical research medical histories.

Eleven years following the establishment of the SPC, the Jesuits established their own Medical School of St. Joseph University. A healthy rivalry began between the two institutions, which has flourished into the twenty-first century. Furthermore, the graduate physicians of the Faculty of Medicine of the AUB were looked on by the French medical faculty counterpart as relying on clinical laboratory testing to verify or complement the clinical diagnosis of disease. The French medical faculty graduates were mainly clinicians, using a certain "clinical sense" to arrive at a diagnosis. Though they utilized the laboratory, over the years the laboratory testing was used with equal emphasis for diagnostic purposes. Although secondary to their clinical sense, the French-educated doctors utilized the laboratory with equal emphasis as the American-educated physicians.

My purpose here is to document the origins of medical research and its emerging importance equal to the high quality of education at AUB, as well as to include my experience in medical research.

CHAPTER 2

SECTION 1: Selected Individual Faculty Achievements in the Faculty of Medicine of the American University of Beirut

This chapter discusses the foundation for medical education papers of the faculty of the SPC, with bibliography, covering the period 1920–1974. There are two exceptions of scientific research prior to 1920: the scientific work of Dr. George Post on the classification of the flora of Lebanon, Syria, and Palestine; and his classification and treatment of renal calculosis and an important discussion of the experiments of Dr. Harris Graham on dengue fever, which may be viewed as the earliest basic scientific research.

Interspersed with the above narrative is my own information (which I have included as reflections) on my grandfather Jirius Nassar (BS 1878), along with other Nassar relatives and family friends. Those reflections, though not in the domain of medical research, emphasize the excellent educational attributes of the medical education at the SPC and the AUB.

Historical perspectives of medical education are gleaned from published reports of the SPC 1866–1920. For the sake of educating physicians enrolled in the department of medicine at the SPC, Dr. Cornelius Van Dyck, an 1839 graduate of Jefferson Medical College in Philadelphia, Pennsylvania, and a medical scholar and a linguist with knowledge of several languages, embarked on writing in Arabic and translating English texts to Arabic. He published the following educational texts. (These are included to show the power of the written word, but they by no means can be classified as clinical research.)

- three elementary textbooks of mathematics
- two texts on astronomy
- five chemistry texts
- *Principles of Diagnosis*
- *Principles of Pathology*

He also wrote several other articles and texts not related to medical teaching or research.

An excellent teacher, Dr. Van Dyck taught clinical medicine and ophthalmology. In addition, assisted by Nassif al Yazigi and Butrus Bustani, he completed the translation of the Bible from English to Arabic. The translation began as a lifetime pursuit/work by Reverend Ely Smith (1801–1857), and it was completed after his death.

The next important educational texts were undertaken by Dr. George E. Post, a graduate of the University College of New York, with surgical specialty. He published eighteen articles in Arabic, and at least two texts published in Arabic to English, one of which was a revised second edition of an important reference work for educational purposes.

- *Arabic Dictionary of the Holy Bible*[4]
- "Battle of Encounter at Asus"[5]
- "Classification and Analysis of Stones," *Physician News* [Nassar comment: Urologic document bordering on early clinical pathology of urinary calculi, a valuable reference for physicians]
- "Classification and Study of Principles of Plant Physiology and Function" (can be considered a textbook classifying plants; published in Arabic in 1881)[6]
- "Destruction of Urinary Stones and Their Removal in One Sitting" (again, an educational clinical application for treating urinary calculi)[7]
- *The Flora of Syria, Palestine and Sinai* (an enlarged edition from the original Arabic text of Dr. G. Post), edited by John E. Dinsmore[8]
- *Healthy Medical Upbringing*[9]
- *Index of the Holy Bible*[10]
- "The Order of the Human Vertebral Column" (eight articles in Arabic), *Physician News*, Beirut,1882
- "The Plague"[11]
- *Plantae Postiannae*[12]
- *Plant Science*[13]
- "Plants in Syria and Palestine"[14]
- "Plants of the Near East"[15]
- "Rules How to Succeed"[16]
- "Taxonomy of Plants of Syria and Egypt"[17]

---

4   George E. Post, *Arabic Dictionary of the Holy Bible* (Beirut, Lebanon: American Press, 1894).

5   George E. Post, "Battle of Encounter at Asus," *At Tabib* newspaper (November 1881): 376–379, 391–394.

6   George E. Post, "Classification and Study of Principles of Plant Physiology and Function" (Arabic) (Beirut, Lebanon, 1881).

7   George E. Post, "Destruction of Urinary Stones and Their Removal in One Sitting," *At Tabib* newspaper (March 1881): 62–65.

8   George E. Post, *The Flora of Syria, Palestine and Sinai* (Beirut, Lebanon: American Press, 1932).

9   George E. Post, *Healthy Medical Upbringing* (Arabic) (Beirut, Lebanon, 1881).

10   George E. Post, *Index of the Holy Bible* (Arabic) (Beirut, Lebanon, 1873).

11   George E. Post, "The Plague," *At Tabib* newspaper (May 1881): 83–87.

12   George E. Post, *Plantae Postiannae* (Lausanne, Switzerland: Bridel, 1890).

13   George E. Post, *Plant Science* (Arabic) (Beirut, Lebanon, 1881).

14   George E. Post, "Plants in Syria and Palestine," *Al-Muktataf* 8 (1883): 417–422.

15   George E. Post, "Plants of the Near East," *Al-Muktataf* 8 (1883): 81–83.

16   George E. Post, "Rules How to Succeed," *Al-Muktataf* 6 (1881): 215–219, 276–273.

17   George E. Post, "Taxonomy of Plants of Syria and Egypt," *At Tabib* newspaper (August 1883): 211–213.

- "Terpentina in Cancer"[18]
- "Treatment of Acute Intestinal Obstruction Using 'Affuwn,'" *Physician Newspaper* (February 1881): 46–49.

The above cited bibliography is my own translation of the references into English. The published work of *The Flora of Syria, Palestine and Sinai*, though its core is taxonomy, it may be considered perhaps the earliest scientific reference textbook of the college for students of botany, and a pharmaceutical source. It is of interest to me personally to note that its publication in Arabic was with the assistance of my grandfather, Jirius Nassar (BS 1878), who was Dr. Post's student and colleague friend.

Under the leadership of Reverend Daniel Bliss, and his son, Howard Bliss, and also Dr. Cornelius Van Dyck, with Dr. G. E. Post of the Medical Department, and later in 1915 with Dr. William Van Dyck and other notable physicians, the Syrian Protestant College's medical department became top-notch, excelling in medical education and graduating many distinguished physicians. However, medical research was shrouded in medical education, for several reasons:

- In the early history of the medical department of the Syrian Protestant College, the available educational funds were sufficient to teach and educate students in languages, literature, and in medicine and the sciences. No funds were available for medical clinical research or otherwise.
- The sociocultural atmosphere of the Near East communities was directed mostly toward education and important religious beliefs. Research was unheard of at the time. Secular educational policy was limited by the atmosphere of sectarian communities. Due to the influence of a cultural mix of religions, embarking on medical research would have been counter to the beliefs prevailing at that time of an awakening in medical education.
- A crisis in the medical department developed on July 19, 1882, following Dr. Edwin Lewis's address to the graduating class. Dr. Lewis mentioned Darwin and Pasteur, implying (my own opinion) that students develop an inquisitive approach to science and to new theories. Such implications did not sit well with the conservative Board of Commission Managers, who asked Dr. Lewis to resign. Subsequently, Dr. C. Van Dyck left the Department of Medicine, with some student followers, in protest to the action of the board. Two authors wrote about the "crisis." First, Professor Shafiq Geha, a historian, wrote a book in Arabic and later on published in English, titled *Darwin and the Crisis of 1882 in the Medical Department of the Syrian Protestant College* (AUB Press, 2004). Second, Dr. Farid S. Haddad also mentioned Professor Geha's work and in a scholarly fashion evaluated the "crisis" in his published book about the life of his

---

18   George E. Post, "Terpentina in Cancer," *At Tabib* newspaper (December 1881): 16.

father, entitled *A First-Class Man in Every Particular: Dr. Sami I. Haddad (1890–1957)*, (Shad Board AZ, USA, 2001), 85.

Although the talent and ability of the physician graduates and the excellence in educating them was ever present, medical research gradually became established, slowly but surely, due to the genius of the AUB Faculty of Medicine and its graduates that outshone the lack of funding for research. Such a trend toward clinical (and to a certain extent, scientific preclinical) research began to appear from 1920 and beyond. The extent to which Dr. Lewis's mention of Darwin influenced the student body of SPC and AUB in 1920 and beyond remains a matter of conjecture.

[**Nassar comment:** A special mention is made here of Dr. Harris Graham, who probably was the first SPC physician-pathologist to do basic scientific research on dengue fever as early as 1898. Dr. Graham noted prior epidemics of dengue fever in Europe and similar manifestation of symptoms and signs of dengue that were prevalent in Beirut and nearby areas (fever, joint pains, prostration with skin rashes or hemorrhages). His research was published in the *Journal of Tropical Medicine* dated July 1903, pp. 210–214. He made astute clinical observations gathered on dengue fever cases in men and adolecents infected by the mosquito Culex Fatigans. He also inoculated volunteers with the dengue fever mosquito and reported on their clinical illness. He postulated that the mosquito transmitted the infection of parasitic particles that invaded red blood corpuscles similar to malarial infestation. At one point in the written text of the article, he mentions the word *virus*. Modern medicine now has isolated a flaviuvirus as the culprit transmitted by the mosquito. A. Egyptei]. (Ref. B. K. Mandal and colleagues, "Dengue Fever," *Lecture Notes on Infectious Diseases*, 5th ed. (UK: Blakwell Sciences Ltd., 1996), 303-330)

Several physicians should be mentioned who contributed to clinical published reports that may have stimulated clinical and/or basic research. One of these was Dr. Nimeh Nucho, professor emeritus of chest diseases, who in 1911 wrote the article "Medical Notes: Observations on the Importance of a Microscopic Examination in the Diagnosis and Treatment of Tumors."[19] This paper emphasized the importance of identifying tumors by their pathology. He drew the attention of the practicing physicians at the time to the pathology of tumors and their importance in their clinical diagnosis.

Dr. Nucho became very famous in his diagnosis and treatment of tuberculosis, and he headed the Hamlin Hospital in the mountains near Hamana Village. The Hamlin Hospital, also known as Chbaniyeh, was founded by Mary Eddy and the Quakers. After the tragic death of Dr. Nucho, his son, Dr. Charles Khalil Nucho, assumed the directorship of the hospital.

---

19   Nemeh Nucho, "Medical Notes: Observations on the Importance of a Microscopic Examination in the Diagnosis and Treatment of Tumors," *Al-Kulliyeh* III (1911): 63–66.

Another paper in Arabic by Dr. Nehme Nucho, most interestingly, was on the treatment of malignant pleural effusion using the surgical method of pleurodesis. This treatment, which currently uses cyclosporine or talcum powder injected into the pleural space to prevent pleural fluid from reaccumulating, could have been a prologue for research assessing its long-term effectiveness in preventing pleural effusion recurrence [*Al-Kulliyeh* (1928): 129–136].

Dr. Harris Graham wrote an article entitled "Medical Notes. A New Typhoid Serum."[20] This paper would nowadays have alerted pharmaceutical companies to start research to find and produce other typhoid vaccines for the prevention of typhoid infectious disease. Currently there are three inactivated parenteral typhoid vaccines and one live attenuated vaccine given orally (*ACP Task Force on Adult Immunization and Infectious Diseases Society of America*, 3rd edition, 1994).

Another important work of Dr. Graham was probably among the first published papers that truly was the first basic scientific research worked up and written in the *Journal of Tropical Medicine* titled, "Dengue: A Study of Its Propagation and Mode of Propagation" (July 1, 1903): 209–214.

Dr. Harry G. Dorman wrote three significant articles:

- "Medical Notes. A Case Report of Traumatic Popliteal Aneurism."[21] This report, to a research-minded surgeon, may point to the importance of vascular medicine-surgery in peripheral arterial disease.
- "Medical Notes. The Open Reduction Treatment of Fractures."[22] Though educational in the subject matter, it does point to further double-blind studies versus closed reduction to verify its significance.
- With Dr. P. F. Sahyoun, "Identification and Significance of Spirochetes in the Placenta."[23] This work is very significant because it proved that spirochetes cross the placenta to the fetus, a fact that was not clearly established in the medical community worldwide. This is the cause for congenital syphilis.

Faris Sahyoun (MD, SPC, 1875) wrote two volumes of pharmacology (source, Dr. Farid S. Haddad), an example of unpublished achievement reference.

---

20   Harris Graham, "Medical Notes. A New Typhoid Serum," *Al-Kulliyeh* II (1911): 264–266.

21   Harry G. Dorman, "Medical Notes. A Case Report of Traumatic Popliteal Aneurism," *Al-Kulliyeh* II (1911): 306–316.

22   Harry G. Dorman, "Medical Notes. The Open Reduction Treatment of Fractures," *Al-Kulliyeh* IV (1913): 223–225.

23   Harry G. Dorman and P. F. Sahyoun, "Identification and Significance of Spirochetes in the Placenta," *American Journal of Obstetrics & Gynecology* XXXIII (1937): 954–967.

Dr. John Wortabet ...

- wrote *Clarification of Anatomical Dissection* (Beirut, 1871): 7,421 pages[24]
- translated "Principles of Physiology," by Criks and Baker, to Arabic (Beirut, 1877): 65 pages
- translated "Physiology Atlas and Dissection," by Turner, to Arabic (Beirut, 1881)
- coauthored with Rev. Harvey Porter *Arabic-English, English-Arabic Dictionary* (1954)[25]

Dr. Wortabet also authored several articles in Arabic dealing with health education and healthy living, the emphasis being on educating the public.

The period 1900–1920 witnessed several prominent American and Lebanese physicians, both from the faculty and graduates of SPC, who primarily wrote educational medical articles in Arabic and English. Again, the emphasis was on teaching undergraduate and graduate medical doctors. The American faculty were:

- Dr. Franklin Moore, who headed the Department of Obstetrics-Gynecology;
- Dr. Charles A. Webster, who headed the Department of ENT;
- Dr. Edwin St. John Ward, dean of the medical school, who headed the Department of Surgery, following the retirement of Dr. G. E. Post in 1907–1908; and
- Dr. William Van Dyck, who took over the duties of Dr. Dorman, who took over Dr. Moore's department in 1915.

The following are some prominent Lebanese physicians. (I ask the reader's permission to digress from the theme of this book, my justification being to enlighten the reader of some biography about important faculty of medicine, whose work may or may not be on clinical research.)

- Dr. Nemeh Nucho, born 1903. Dr. Nucho was professor of chest disease and later on professor emeritus from 1949–1954. He was director and physician in-chief of Hamlin Hospital Sanatorium for TB, Hammana, Lebanon.
- Dr. Sami I. Haddad, born 1890, faculty, MD SPC 1913. Dr. Haddad was the first Lebanese physician surgeon to become Fellow of the FACS in 1934, and the first Lebanese to be professor of surgery in 1939 and dean of the School of Medicine (now Faculty of Medicine) of the American University of Beirut. He was a brilliant surgeon and physician, renowned in the Middle East, and a promoter of the history of Arab medicine (collected 125 Arab medical manuscripts) and its physicians' contributions to medicine, including medical-surgical research. His son, Dr. Farid S. Haddad, wrote

---

24 *Clarification of Anatomical Dissection* (Beirut, Lebanon, 1871).
25 John Wortabet and Harvey Porter, *Arabic-English, English-Arabic Dictionary* (1954).

a fascinating biography of his life and work. Dr. Sami I. Haddad was the first to introduce cystoscopy, and among few physicians in the Middle East to research the lives and contributions of Arab physicians and their discoveries. His research included Ibn An Nafis and his discovery of the "pulmonary circulation of the blood," which refuted Galen's work, and predated the research work of Dr. William Harvey and his description of the circulation of the blood and heart "motion" by at least three hundred years. Dr. Sami I. Haddad wrote seventy-four medical articles in various local and international journals, as well as on original works of Arab doctors, which have been collated by Dr. Farid S. Haddad in the Sami I. Haddad Library.

- Dr. Amin A. Khairallah was on the faculty from 1933–1955. He was an excellent surgeon and director of the National Hospital, better known as Khairallah Hospital. He published twelve articles, the first three in Arabic. He also collaborated with Dr. Sami Haddad, who wrote "Discoverer of the Lessor Circulation of the Blood" (refer to chapter 4).

≠ "A Century of American Medicine in Syria"[26]

≠ "Importance of Social Medicine and Its Goals"[27]

≠ "Investigation of the Gall Bladder"[28]

≠ *La convalescence chirurgical, Rev. Med. Moy. Or.* IV (1947): 599

≠ *Le traitement des chole'cystites, Rev. Med. Moy. Or.* (1948) : 411–419

≠ "Malaria Prevention in the Beka' Valley"[29]

≠ "Outline of Arabic Contributions to Medicine and the Allied Sciences"[30]

≠ "The Significance of Arabic Culture"[31]

≠ "Some Cultural Aspects of Medical History and Literature"[32]

≠ "Some Historical Outlook of Medicine and Its Ethical Culture"[33]

≠ "Some Rarer Manifestations of Chronic Appendicitis"[34]

---

26   Amin A. Khairallah, "A Century of American Medicine in Syria," *American Medical History* 1 (1939): 460–470.

27   Amin A. Khairallah, "Importance of Social Medicine and Its Goals," *Al Abhath* (June 3, 1950): 205–215.

28   Amin A. Khairallah, "Investigation of the Gall Bladder," *Journal Palestine Arab Medical Association* 1 (1946): 38.

29   Amin A. Khairallah, "Malaria Prevention in the Beka'a Plain," *Al Majalah Tibiah Al Elmiyah* (August 1947).

30   Amin A. Khairallah, "Outline of Arabic Contributions to Medicine and the Allied Sciences," (Beirut, Lebanon: American Press, 1946).

31   Amin A. Khairallah, "The Significance of Arabic Culture," *Al Kulliyah Review* (April 1946).

32   Amin A. Khairallah, "Some Cultural Aspects of Medical History and Literature," *Journal Palestine Arab Medical Association* 2 (1947): 38.

33   Amin A. Khairallah, "Some Historical Outlook of Medicine and Its Ethical Culture," *Al Majalah Tibiah Al Ilmiyah* (August 1947).

34   Amin A. Khairallah, "Some Rarer Manifestations of Chronic Appendicitis," *Journal Palestine Arab Medical Association* 2 (1946): 38.

≠ "A Study of Arab Hospitals in the Light of Present Day Standardization"[35] (Standardization of health care in US hospitals began in 1910, by Dr. Ernst Codman. It was the early start of the Joint Commission for Accreditation of Hospitals.)

- Dr. Yusif Hitti, an excellent internist and head of the German Hospital. Following his graduation with the MD (SPC 1917), he trained in internal medicine at Harvard Medical School. He was then appointed professor of anatomy and internal medicine at AUB until 1928, whereupon he accepted the directorship of St. Charles Boromé Hospital (the German Hospital in Beirut). He wrote papers on the incidence of the disease kala azar in infants and in adults in Syria. He also wrote on the fever treatment of syphilis of the CNS, many years ahead of the discovery of penicillin and its treatment. In 1967, Dr. Yusif Hitti wrote a monumental medical Arabic-English dictionary, three editions (with the assistance of my uncle, Fuad Jirius Nassar, an expert in the Arabic language, as well as author of several books in Arabic). He also translated into Arabic H. T. Hyman's *The Complete Home Medical Encyclopedia*. He also served as head of the Department of Makassed Hospital 1950–1958. He was awarded the Order of Commander of the British Empire, the Daniel Bliss Gold Medal, and the AUB Alumni Gold Medal. It is of interest to note that the parents of brothers Phillip and Yusif Hitti, who lived in Chemlan village west of Souk El Gharb, were cajoled and enticed by my grandfather, Jirius Nassar (BS, SPC 1878), to enroll their children in Souk El Gharb high school where he was principal. They excelled and were admitted to the SPC following their high school graduation. Dr. Yusif Hitti graduated with an MD degree in 1917. Dr. Phillip Hitti specialized in Arab history and Semitic languages and became professor emeritus at Princeton University. Among his many writings about Arab scholars, he included Ibn An Nafis, with the latter's contribution in "Sharh Tashrih al-Quanun, a Clear Concept of the Pulmonary Circulation." Professor Hitti, and one famous US surgeon, Dr. Cruikshank, on a pilgrimage, visited Ibn Sina's gravesite.[36]
- Dr. Jabra Obeid, a brilliant diagnostician, internist-generalist. He saved my life as a three-year-old boy with typhoid fever. Dr. Obeid graduated with the MD degree from AUB in 1922. He was an example of the strength of medical education at AUB.
- Dr. Fayez S. Nassar, MD, 1911, a pioneer military physician, worked in Khartoum, Sudan. He enlisted in the Anglo-Egyptian army with the rank of colonel. He became a tropical disease expert at the military hospital, especially on sleeping sickness and black water fever. He was bestowed the title of Bey by the British-Egyptian authorities, the Commander of the British Empire Medal was bestowed upon him by the King of England, and the coveted Medal of the Nile was given to him by the Egyptian

---

35 Amin A. Khairallah and S. I. Haddad, "A Study of Arab Hospitals in the Light of Present Day Standardization," *Bulletin: American College of Surgeons* XXI (1936): 173.

36 Philip Hitti, *History of the Arabs, Revised: 10th Edition* (Palgrave Macmillan, September 6, 2002), 54.

government for medical services rendered to the troops. Hunting big game was his hobby, and in his retirement he wrote a book on hunting, relating his experiences.[37]

- Dr. Halim Saadeh, MD, 1911, almost failed to graduate; however, he also joined the Egyptian Army and reached the rank of colonel. He was a good family physician. He saved my life at age four years. At that time, the AUB Hospital refused his request to admit me for treatment with the diphtheria antitoxin. Throughout his professional life he was bitter toward AUB. His wife suffered from rheumatic heart disease. When she had a turn for the worse, he asked me, a medical student at the time, to obtain for him Dr. Paul Dudley White's textbook on heart disease from the library. I relate this personal event to show the strength of education at AUB in building strong character and self-reliance, and the unpleasant relationship between Dr. Saadeh and AUB.

- Dr. Franklin Moore wrote several "Medical Notes" in the *Al-Kulliyeh* magazine from 1911 through 1914, including a paper on medical ethics that may be considered a first, again, with emphasis on education. Dr. Moore was very well liked. He passed away prematurely in 1915. Medical ethics and social aspects of medicine (the humanities) were unknown in the region.

- Dr. Webster wrote a few papers dealing with social aspects of medicine in the *Al-Kulliyeh* magazine from 1911 through 1914.

- Dr. Edwin St. John Ward wrote six articles in Arabic published in *Al-Kulliyeh* dealing with medical education and the use of roentgen rays in the diagnosis of disease. Also, he wrote three articles in English published in *Al-Kulliyeh*, one on a trip to Cilicia, another about surgery and the use of anesthesia, and lastly, about the place of the physician graduate in the new era.

In conclusion, 621 physicians were graduated in comparison to 280 published articles, textbooks, and reports in the same period.

---

37   Fayez S. Nassar, *Memoirs of the Sudan* (Beirut, Lebanon: Rihani House Publications Beirut, 1963).

SECTION 2: Birth of Basic Scientific Clinical Papers and Research of the Faculty of Medicine of the American University of Beirut, 1920–1974: Medical History in the Making

The rich heritage of Arabian medicine stemming from the Middle East needs reemphasis. It became established through famous physicians before the rise of Islam and afterward, and continued through the Dark Ages on to the twenty-first century. It is an established, credible fact that the Arab scholars preserved the rich heritage of astronomy, algebra, languages, history, mathematics, medicine, poetry, religion, and social culture during the Dark Ages of Europe, and that without this effort, Europe would have remained unenlightened for many years [J. R. Hayes, ed., *The Genius of Arab Civilization Source of Renaissance*, 2nd edition (Cambridge, MA: MIT Press, 1983)]. The history of Arab medicine and its physicians deserves another write-up in book form and is not included in this manuscript, though its rich heritage may have influenced the writings of clinical reports of physicians of SPC and AUB. Hence, included here are several references on Arab medicine. Those references may not have basic research; however, they were the foundation of clinical research for future generations to rely on, such as what the future history revealed at the SPC and the Faculty of Medicine of AUB.

Furthermore, for the reader interested in pursuing the known writings of Arab physicians, I have included here important references as follows:

- Dr. Farid Sami Haddad wrote extensively on the subject of the legacy of Arab contributions to the field of medicine. Here is an example: "Pioneers of Arabian Medicine," *Leb. Med. J.* (1968), 21: 67–80, with several references.

  ≠ *Al-Kulliyah Rev.* 4 (1937): 1
  ≠ *Ann. Hist. Med.* 3 (1941): 60
  ≠ *The Ann. Rep. Orient Hosp.* 14 (1961): 28
  ≠ "Arab Contribution to Medicine," *Leb. Med. J.* 26:4 (1973): 331–346
  ≠ Browne, *Arabian Medicine* (Cambridge, 1921), 126
  ≠ Campbell, *Arabian Medicine*, 2 vols. (London, 1926)
  ≠ Comston, *An Introduction to the History of Medicine* (London, 1926)
  ≠ C. A. Elgood, *Medical History of Persia and the Eastern Caliphate* (Cambridge, 1957)
  ≠ Grinner, *The Canon of Avicenna* (London, 1930)
  ≠ *Ann. Rep. Orient Hosp.* 14:73 (1961), 15:45 (1962), 18:80 (1965)
  ≠ *Ann. Surg. Bull. A.C.S.* 104:1, 21:173 (1936)

≠ "History of Medicine in Lebanon" (in Arabic), *Leb. Med. J.* 21 (1968): 1–4

≠ Keys & Wakim, *Proc. St. Mect. Mayo Cl.* 28:423 (1953)

≠ L. Leclerc, *La médecine arabe* (1876)

≠ Near East Colleges, 19:1 (1929)

≠ The Near East, 8:12 (1955)

≠ L. Sa'di, *Ann. Med. Hist.* 7:62 (1935)

≠ G. Sarton, *Introduction of the History of Science*, 4 vols.

≠ M. S. Spink, *Proc. Roy. Soc. Med.* 553 (1937)

≠ "The History of Urology in the Middle East."

≠ Proceedings of the First International Congress on "History Knowledge and Quality of Life in Urology" (Fuggi, 1992): 1008–1011, ed., Marandola pp. 41–48. (This paper is an excellent historical review of the onset of modern urological practice in the Arab world: Lebanon, Syria, Palestine, Jordan, Iraq, Kuwait, Arabia, Egypt, and lately to include Iran, Afghanistan, the Arabian Peninsula, The Emirates, Bahrain, Oman, Qatar, the Sudan, and sub-Saharan Africa. It includes forty-four references.)

In his paper, "The History of Urology," Dr. Farid S. Haddad starts with the urological diseases prevalent from prebiblical times on to the classical period. These include …

- Sumerian urology: The library of Ashurbanipal contained nine hundred of three thousand clay tablets that dealt with medicine dating to around 4,000 BC, including a Sumerian dictionary dating back to 4,000 BC, which mentions anatomical parts of the body including the kidney and genitals. Physicians used a catheter to treat gonorrhea [J. Bitschai and M. Brodny, *A History of Urology in Egypt* (Riverside Press, 1956)], and they used belladonna to treat bladder spasm. They also mentioned impotence.

- Egyptian urology: In 1901, the archeologist G. Elliot Smith discovered a tomb of a sixteen-year-old boy who had a vesicle calculus. Its structure was described by Shattuck and the stone was placed in the Royal College of Surgeons in London. Information of Egyptian knowledge of urology comes from two papyri:

  ≠ The Georg Ebers papyrus copy dating to around 1,552 BC, which is now in a medical library in Leipzig, Germany.

  ≠ The Edwin Smith papyrus excavated in 1862 and found at Thebes. Those papyri showed that the Egyptians had knowledge that dislocation of the cervical spine, reported on three of forty-eight cases, had resulted in erection and seminal emission. They also showed hemorrhage following circumcision, and the finding of hydrocele (Morton, Bitschai). Also mentioned were urinary retention, bed-wetting, cystitis, priapism, gonorrhea, and impotence (Worth).

  ≠ Also, the Berlin papyrus of 1,300 BC described the prediction of the sex of the unborn baby using wheat and barley watered daily by the urine of the pregnant woman: If wheat grew, it was a boy and for barley, it was a girl. It is of interest to note that Ibn abi Usaibia described the same test 2,500 years later.

Modern urology in Lebanon: It can be emphatically stated that it was ushered in and pioneered by Dr. Sami I. Haddad (1890–1957). After his graduation from the American University of Beirut School of Medicine, he was awarded a Rockefeller Scholarship for specialization in urology at Johns Hopkins with the father of American urology, Hugh Hampton Young (1921–1922) (Haddad, 1990). He performed the first cystoscopy as a Lebanese physician in 1923. In 1937, he was the surgery professor at the Faculty of Medicine of AUB, and in 1941, the dean of the faculty. He was a staunch leader of the faculty during that difficult period in Lebanon during WWII.

Dr. Sami I. Haddad was a man of great achievements in medicine, unequaled at the time. In 1947, he founded his private not-for-profit hospital, the Orient Hospital in Beirut, with its famous publication, the *Annual Report of the Orient Hospital* (AROH).

Dr. Haddad's surgical firsts are memorable. For the reader of the history of Middle Eastern medicine in the 1920s through the 1940s, there were no first achievements recorded that denoted progress in surgical procedures, except those by Dr. Sami I. Haddad: those achievements are recorded by Dr. Farid S. Haddad as reference.

Dr. Farid S. Haddad (MD 1948), "like father like son," continued the modern progress of urology in Lebanon with many noteworthy accomplishments. He was the first to introduce endoscopic urology-transurethral resection of enlarged prostate in the Middle East, as well as the first to introduce aortography, arteriography, vesiculography, lymphography, and retroperitoneal oxygen insufflation. In 1957, Dr. Haddad founded the Urological Society of Lebanon. He was its first president, and he continued in that position for the subsequent ten years (1957–1967). In 1964, with the collaboration of Dr. Emile Bitar, Dr. Farid S. Haddad founded the Society of the History of Medicine of Lebanon.

In his book, *Two Score and Ten Years of Urology*, published by Shad Broad (2002, 432 pages), Dr. Farid S. Haddad discusses his years of urological and surgical experiences with many firsts in discoveries, case reports, and treatments. It is a modern text of urology, for study by generations of students of urology.

These were most extraordinary achievements, all with distinction. He set an example very difficult to follow both in medical research and as an educator, a product of the American University of Beirut Faculty of Medicine and of his mentors and teachers of the specialty of urology at Chicago's Presbyterian Hospital, Memorial Hospital, and Sloan Kettering Institute, as well by his dad, Dr. Sami I. Haddad.

References:

- Farid S. Haddad, "Analysis of the First Five Thousand Admissions to the Orient Hospital," *Annual Report of the Orient Hospital (AROH)* 8:3–13–17 (1955).
- Farid S. Haddad, *AROH* 10 (1957): 9–10, 12, 16; also Directory of Fellowship awards for the years 1917–1950, Rockefeller Foundation, *AROH* 22 (1969): 26.
- Farid S. Haddad and Sami I. Haddad, "Patellectomy in the Treatment of Fractures of the Patella," *AROH* 3 (1950): 38–51; and *Albustan* (Paradise Valley, AZ, 2006): 153–166.
- Farid S. Haddad and Sami I. Haddad, "Gall Bladder Disease," *AROH* 16 (1969, 1963): 1193–1195; and *Albustan* (Paradise Valley, AZ, 2006): 81–88–90 (lumbar cholecystectomy).
- Farid S. Haddad, BA, MD, FACS, DABU, KNOC, ONOC, CNOC, *Annotated and Illustrated Bibliography*, The Sami I. Haddad Memorial Library Shad Board (2007).
- Farid S. Haddad, Fuad N. Haddad, and Sami I. Haddad, "Remote Metastases from Laryngeal Cancer," and *Albustan* (Paradise Valley, AZ, 2006): 257–259.
- Farid S. Haddad, et al., "Volvulus of the Intestines," *AROH* 14 (1961): 5–12; and *Albustan* (Paradise Valley, AZ, 2006): 171–176, 178.
- Sami I. Haddad, "100 Cases Submitted to the ACS" (1934, unpublished); and *Albustan* (Paradise Valley, AZ, 2006): 56, 59–60.
- Sami I. Haddad, "Essentials of Urinary and Genital Diseases" (Beirut: American Press, 1946).
- Sami I. Haddad, "Hydatid Disease of the Lungs," *AROH* 1 (1948): 49–53.
- Farid S. Haddad and Sami I. Haddad, "Hydatid Diseases in the Lebanon," *AROH* (1949): 102-282; and *Albustan* (Paradise Valley, AZ, 2006): 104–122.
- Sami I. Haddad, "The Surgical Treatment of 'Nodular' Lung Disease" (translated from Arabic), *AROH* 3 (1950): 37–47.
- Sami I. Haddad, "Thoracoplasty in the Treatment of Pulmonary Tuberculosis," *AROH* 3 (1950): 52–62.
- Sami I. Haddad, "Elephantiasis," *AROH* 4 (1951): 83–85, and *Albustan* (Paradise Valley, AZ, 2006): 167–169.
- Sami I. Haddad, "Foreign Bodies in the Esophagus," *AROH* 7 (1954): 43, and *Albustan* (Paradise Valley, AZ, 2006), 138–139.
- Sami I. Haddad and Farid S. Haddad, "Surgery of the Vegetative Nervous System," *J. Palest. Arab Med. Ass.* 2 (1947): 63–71, and *Albustan* (Paradise Valley, AZ, 2006), 141–149.
- Sami I. Haddad and Fuad S. Haddad, "Carcinoma of the Rectum and Its Operative Treatment," *AROH* 3 (1950): 20–31, and *Albustan* (Paradise Valley, AZ, 2006): 303, 313–314.
- Sami I. Haddad and Fuad S. Haddad, "Retropubic Prostatectomy," 3 (1950): 32–37, and *Albustan* (Paradise Valley, AZ, 2006): 267–373.
- Sami I. Haddad and Amin A. Khairallah, "A Forgotten Chapter in the History of the Circulation of the Blood," *Ann. Surg.* vol. 104 (July 1936): 1–8.
- Sami I. Haddad, "Who Is the Discoverer of the Lesser Circulation," *Muktataf J.* 89 (1936): 264.

CHAPTER 3

Published Preclinical and Clinical Research Papers of the Faculty of Medicine of AUB by Author Department

The following section lists examples of published papers of basic preclinical research and clinical research by departments of the Faculty of Medicine of the American University of Beirut during the golden age period. This is in contradistinction from the published papers by alphabetic names of authors of the Faculties of the University, compiled by Mrs. Suha Tamim (see below).

This manuscript demonstrates medical preclinical and clinical research activity of the Medical Faculty that emerged alongside the medical education of medical students of AUB Faculty of Medicine. Additionally, I have reviewed certain articles of interest to establish documentary evidence of the ongoing research, a type of history in the making, covering the period of 1920–1974.

I hope that the new physician graduates of the Faculty of Medicine would return to the Saab Medical Library and review the medical articles of "old-timers" as a source for their medical research.

The period of 1975–2008 covers a continuation of my journey into medical research which had part of its beginnings during my cardiology fellowships in the United States (see chapter 4).

The list includes the medical research published in the English language. Research papers published in Arabic can be found in *A Bibliography of A.U.B. Faculty Publications 1866–1966* compiled by Mrs. Suha Tamim (Tuqan) for the Centennial Publications of AUB, edited by Dr. Fuad Sarruf. Any omission of research workers in various departments is purely unintentional.

My approach is to comment on examples of one or two published papers from each medical department (or otherwise) proving thus the active research in the golden period of the Faculty of Medicine 1920–1974.

Department of Anatomy and Histology

Afifi, Adil K.

- (with M. W. Shanklin, S. A. Hashim, and N. A. Acra) "Concurrent Demonstration of Desoxyribose Nucleic Acid and 1, 2, Glycols," *Stain Technology*, XXVIII (1953): 113–118.
- (with N. A. Acra) "Concurrent Demonstration of Desoxyribose Nucleic Acid and 1, 2, Glycols 2: Periodate Oxidation," *Stain Technology*, XXX (1955): 119–122.
- (with M. W. Shanklin and A. N. Azzam) "Application of the Periodic Acid Sciff Procedure to Tissue Block," *Stain Technology*, XXXV (1960): 325–330.
- (with K. A. Kurban) "Alkaline Phosphatase Activity in Skin as Shown by Staining en Bloc," *Stain Technology*, XXXVII (1962): 7–11.
- "The Camel Subcommisural Organ," *Journal of Comparative Neurology*, CXXIII (1964): 139–145.

Ghantus, Musa, Chairman and later Dean; 1928–1966

- (with S. E. Kerr and B. F. Avery) "The Lactic Acid Content of Mammalian Brain," *Journal of Biological Chemistry*, CX (1935): 542-637. For comment on papers on brain metabolism, see Dr. Kerr's papers in collaboration with Dr. Ghantus; "Growth of the Shaft of Human Radius and Ulna during First Two Years of Life," *American Journal Roentgenology, Radium Therapy and Nuclear Medicine*, LXV (1951): 784–786.

Hashim, Sami A.; 1950–1952

- "A Survey of Histochemical Methods Used for the Identification of Polysaccharides and their Derivatives," *Acta Anatomica*, XVI (1952): 355–366.
- "Feulgen Hydrolysis with Phosphoric Acid," *Stain Technology*, XXVII (1953): 27–31.
- (with A. N. Acra) "An Improved Lead-Tetraacetic Acid Schiff Procedure," *Stain Technology*, XXVIII (1953): 1–8.

Shanklin, William M.; chairman of Department of Histology; professor emeritus, 1962–1966 [**Nassar comment:** One of the practical contributions of Professor William M. Shanklin with Tamer K. Nassar and M. Issidorides is a scientific approach methodology in developing a staining solution to improve the clarity of granules in neurons, and also its use in showing clearly reticulum in various organs of the human body in normal and in pathological states as viewed under the microscope. The details of their studies and the composition and making the staining solution can be found in American Medical Association, *Archives of Pathology*, vol. 71 (June 1961): 611–614.]

- "The Central System Chameleon Vulgaris," *Acta Zoologica*, XI (1930): 425–490.
- "American University of Beirut, School of Medicine, Department of Histology and Embryology. Methods and Problems of Medical Education," in *Twentieth Series* (New York: The Rockefeller Foundation, 1932).
- "The Comparative Neurology of the Nucleus Opticus Tegmenti with Special Reference to Chameleon Vulgaris," *Acta Zoologica*, XIV (1933): 163–184.
- (with C. U. Ariens Kappers) "The Anthropology of Transjordan Arabs," *Psychiatrische en Neurologishe Bladen* (1934): 280–289.
- "The Cerebella of Three Deep Sea Fish," *Acta Zoologica*, XV (1934): 409–430.
- "On Diencephalic and Mesencephalic Nuclei and Fibre Paths in the Brains of Three Deep-Sea Fish," *Philosophical Transactions of the Royal Society of London. Series B. Biological Sciences*, CCXXIV (1935): 351–419.
- "Blood Grouping of the Rwala Arabs," *Proceedings of the Society for Experimental Biology and Medicine* (NY), XXXII (1935): 745–755.
- "The Anthropology of the Rwala Bedouins," *Journal of the Royal Anthropological Institute*, LXV (1935): 375–390.
- "Blood Grouping of Rwala Bedouin," *Journal of Immunology*, XXIX (1935): 427–433.
- "Anthropology of the Akeydat and the Manaly Bedouin," *American Journal of Physical Anthropology*, XXI (1936): 252-271.
- "Blood Grouping of the Manaly and Akeydat Bedouin," *American Journal of Physical Anthropology*, XXI (1936): 39–48.
- "Polynuclear Court of the Alouites," *Transactions of the Royal Society of Tropical Medicine and Hygiene*, XXX (1936): 173–178.
- (with N. Izzeddin) "Anthropology of the Near East Female," *American Journal of Physical Anthropology*, XXII (1937): 381–415.
- (with H. Cummings) "Dermatoglyphics in Rwala Bedouins," *Human Biology*, IX (1937): 357–365.
- "Anthropometry of the Syrian Males," *Journal of the Royal Anthropological Institute*, LXVIII (1938): 379–414.
- (with H. Cummings) "Dematoglyphics in Peoples of the Near East. I. Lebanese: Mitwali," *American Journal of Physical Anthropology*, XXII (1937): 263–265.
- "Anthropometry of the Syrian Males," *Journal of the Royal Anthropological Institute*, LXVIII (1938): 379–414.
- "Differentiation of Pituicytes in the Human Foetus," *Journal of Anatomy*, LXXIV (1940): 459–463.
- (with J. S. Jessup) "The Hypothalamus of the Coney, Hyrax Syriaca," *Journal of Comparative Neurology*, LXXII (1940): 329–356.
- (with I. Mahfuz) "The Diencephalon of the Coney, Hyrax Syriaca," *Journal of Comparative Neurology*, LXXV (1941): 427–485.
- "On the Presence of Nerve Cells in the Neurohypopysis of the Dog," *Journal of Anatomy*, LXXII (1943): 241–242.

- "The Hortega Silver Carbonate Method for Staining Pituicytes after Paraffin Embedding," *Stain Technology*, XVIII (1943): 87–89.
- "Histogenesis of Pituicytes in the Chick," *Journal of Anatomy*, LXXVIII (1944): 79–93.
- "Histogenesis of the Pig Neurohypophysis," *American Journal of Anatomy*, LXXIV (1944): 327–353.
- "The Development and Histology of Pituitary Concretions in Man," *Anatomical Record*, XCIV (1946): 597–614.
- "On the Presence of Clefts, Fibroid Neuroglia, Neuro-Blast Like Cells and Nerve Cells in the Human Neurohypophysis," *Anatomical Record*, XCVI (1946): 143–164.
- "Anthropometry of Transjordan Bedouin with a Discussion of Their Racial Affinities," *American Journal of Physical Anthropology*, IV (1946): 323–376.
- "On the Origin of Tumorettes in the Human Neurohypophysis," *Anatomical Record*, LXLIX (1947): 297–328.
- "Mesothelial Concretions and Mesothelium in the Human Pituitary," *Anatomical Record*, CII (1948): 77–102.
- "On the Presence of Calcific Bodies, Cartilage, Bone, Follicular Concretions and the So-called Hyaline Bodies in the Human Pituitary," *Anatomical Record*, CII (1948): 469–492.
- "On the Presence of Cysts in the Human Pituitary," *Anatomical Record*, CIV (1949): 379–408.
- "Anthropology of the Near East," *American Near East Society Monograph Series* (1949): 1–10.
- "Some Experimental Approaches to the Cancer Problem," *Revue Médicale Libanaise*, II (1949): 103–104.
- (with A. Y. Djanian and J. M. Butros) "Effect of Tubercle Bacilli Extracts on Induced Tumors of the Rat," *Cancer Research*, IX (1949): 520–525.
- (with T. K. Nassar) "Staining Pineal Parenchyma by a Modified Hortega Method after Paraffin Embedding," *Stain Technology*, XXV (1950): 35–38.
- (with G. Nassar and A. Y. Djanian) "The Etiological Significance of Ergot in the Incidence of Post-Partum Necrosis of the Anterior Pituitary. A Preliminary Report," *American Journal of Obstetrics and Gynecology*, LX (1950): 140–145.
- "The Incidence and Distribution of Cilia in the Human Pituitary with a Description of Micro-Follicular Cysts Derived from Rathke's Cleft," *Acta Anatomica*, XI (1951): 361–382.
- (with D. Kazzaz) "The Coronary Vessels of the Dog Demonstrated by Colored Plastic (Vinyl Acetate) Injections and Corrosion," *Anatomical Record*, CVII (1950): 43–60.
- (with T. K. Nassar) "Staining Neuroglia with Silver Dianminohydroxide after Sensitizing with Sodium Sulfite and Embedding in Paraffin," *Stain Technology*, XXVI (1951): 13–18.

- (with D. Kazzaz) "Comparative Anatomy of the Superficial Vessels of the Mammalian Kidney Demonstrated by Plastic (Vinyl Acetate) Injections and Corrosion," *Journal of Anatomy*, LXXXV (1951): 163–165.
- "The Histogenesis and Histology of an Integumentary Type of Epithelium in the Human Hypophysis," *Anatomical Record*, CIX (1951): 217–232.
- "Lymphocytes and Lymphoid Tissue in the Human Pituitary," *Anatomical Record*, CXI (1951): 177–192.
- "The Origin, Histology and Senescence of Tumorettes in the Human Neurohypophysis," *Acta Anatomica*, XVIII (1953): 1–20.
- (with S. A. Hashim, A. N. Acra, and A. K. Afifi) "Concurrent Demonstration of Desoxyribose Nucleic Acid and 1, 2–Glycols," *Stain Technology*, XXVIII (1953): 113–118.
- "Age Changes in the Histology of the Human Pituitary," *Acta Anatomica*, XIX (1953): 290–304.
- "Anthropological Measurements of the Arab Bedouin with Comments on Their Customs. Summary of a Communication to the Royal Anthropological Institute, June 30, 1953," *Man*, LIII, article 206 (1953): 134.
- (with A. J. Dark) "Two Skulls from Jordan," *Annual Report of the Department of Antiquities of Jordan*, II (1953): 57–61.
- "Argentophilic Cells in the Adenohypophysis," *Anatomical Record*, CXX (1954): 156.
- (with T. K. Nassar) "A Method for the Silver Impregnation of Muller's Fibers in the Retina after Paraffin Embedding with a Description of the Branches of These Fibers," *Acta Anatomica*, XXV (1955): 188–191.
- (with C. D'Angelo) "Changes in the Fibrillar Tissue of the Human Neurohypophysis Associated with Advancing Age," *Anatomical Record*, CXXV (1956): 55–64.
- "The Human Hypophysis in Cases of Burns," *Acta Endocrinologica*, XXI (1956): 1–7.
- (with C. D'Angelo and M. Issidorides) "A Comparative Study of the Staining Reactions of Granules in the Human Neuron," *Journal of Comparative Neurology*, CVI (1956): 478–506.
- (with M. Issidorides and T. K. Nassar) "Neurosecretion on the Human Cerebellum," *Journal of Comparative Neurology*, CVII (1957): 315–338.
- (with T. K. Nassar and M. Issidorides) "Luxol Fast Blue as a Selective Stain for Alpha Cells in the Human Pituitary," *Stain Technology*, XXXIV (1959): 55–58.
- (with M. Issidorides) "New Applications of Luxol Fast Blue and Periodic Acid-Schiff Staining Methods," (abstract), *Anatomical Record*, CXXXIII (1959): 426–442.
- (with T. K. Nassar) "A Preliminary Survey of Some Cytoplasmic Constituents Stained by Luxol Fast Blue," *Acta Anatomica*, XXXVI (1959): 257–264.
- (with T. K. Nassar) "Luxol Fast Blue Combined with the Periodic Acid-Schiff Procedure for Cytological Staining of Kidney," *Stain Technology*, XXXIV (1959): 257–260.
- (with M. Issidorides) "Preliminary Observations on the Histochemistry of Granular Material in the Human Cerebellum, Hypothalamus and Medulla," (abstract), *Journal of Anatomy*, XCIII (1959): 583.

- (with T. K. Nassar and M. Issidorides) "Concentric Layers in the Granules of Human Nervous Lipofuscin Demonstrated by Silver Impregnation," *Stain Technology*, XXXV (1960): 15–18.
- (with M. Issidorides) "The Use of Luxol Fast Blue as a Counter Stain with the Ninhydrin and Alloxan-Schiff Staining Reaction," *Stain Technology*, XXXV (1960): 46.
- (with M. Issidorides) "Observations on Argentophilic Bodies in the Human Choroid Plexus," (abstract), *Anatomical Record*, CXXXVI (1960): 316.
- (with A. K. Afifi and N. A. Azzam) "Application of the Periodic Acid-Schiff Procedure to Tissue Block," *Stain Technology*, XXXV (1960): 325–330.
- (with T. K. Nassar) "A Simplified Silver Impregnation Oxidation Procedure for Staining Reticulum," *Archives of Pathology*, LXXI (1961): 611–614.
- (with M. Issidorides) "Histochemical Reactions of Cellular Inclusions in the Human Neuron," *Journal of Anatomy*, XCV (1961): 151.
- (with M. Issidorides and N. A. Azzam) "Histochemistry of the Human Choroid Plexus," *Anatomical Record*, CLXI (1961): 21–30.
- "Myelin Figures Demonstrated with the Phase Microscope," *Stain Technology*, XXXVI (1961): 377–378.
- (with M. Issidorides and M. Salam) "Histochemistry of the Cerebral Cortex from a Case of Amaurotic Family Idiocy," *Journal of Neuropathology and Experimental Neurology*, XXI (1962): 284–293.
- (with M. Salam) A Comparison of the Histochemistry of the Cerebral Cortex from Siblings with Gargoylism and Tay-Sach's Disease," *Acta Neurovegetativa*, XXV (1963): 297–309.
- (with C. Mytilineou and M. Issidorides) "Histochemical Reactions of Human Autonomic Ganglia," *Journal of Anatomy*, XCVII (1963): 533–542.
- (with N. A. Azzam) "On the Presence of Valves in the Rat Cerebral Arteries," *Anatomical Record*, CXLVI (1963): 145–148.
- (with N. A. Azzam) "A Study of Valves in the Arteries of the Rodent Brain," *Anatomical Record*, CXLVI (1963): 407–414.
- (with N. A. Azzam) "Phase-Constant Microscopy Applied to PAS-Stained Ground Substance," *Stain Technology*, XXXIX (1964): 110–111.
- (with N. A. Azzam) "Histological and Histochemical Studies on the Incisures of Schmidt-Lanterman," *Journal of Comparative Neurology*, CXXIII (1964): 5–10.
- (with R. H. Brownson and D. B. Suter) "A Study in Chronic Brain Radionecrosis," *Journal of Neuropathology and Experimental Neurology*, CXXIII (1964): 660–675.
- (with N. A. Azzam) "Application of Phase-Contrast Microscopy to Schiff-Positive Material," *Stain Technology*, (in press).

Department of Anesthesiology

Brandstater, Bernard J.; chairman of Anesthesiology Department, 1958–1969

- "Prolonged Intubation: An Alternative to Tracheostomy in Infants," *Proceedings of the First European Congress of Anesthesiology*, (1962): 106.
- "Death from Oxygen Therapy," *Lancet*, II (1962): 1059.
- (with E. I. Eger) "Solubility of Methoxyflurane in Rubber," *Anesthesiology*, XXIV (1963): 679–683.
- (with E. I. Eger and G. Edelist) "Controlled-Depth Anesthesia for Respiratory Studies," *Physiologist*, VI (1963): 145.
- (with J. W. Severinghaus, E. I. Eger, and H. Chiodi) "Cerebral Blood Flow in Chronic Hypoxia," *Acta Anaesthesiologica Scandinavica*, suppl. XV (1964): 96.
- (with E. I. Eger and G. Edelist) "Constant-Depth Halothane Anesthesia in Respiratory Studies," *Journal of Applied Physiology*, XX (1965): 171–174.
- (with E. I. Eger and G. Edelist) "Effects on Respiration of Halothane, Ether and Cyclopropane on Respiration," *British Journal of Anesthesiology*, XXXVII (1965): 890–897.
- (with E. I. Eger and L. Saidman) "Minimum Alveolar Anesthetic Concentration (MAC); A Standard of Anesthetic Potency," *Anesthesiology*, XXVI (1965): 756–763. [**Nassar Comment:** In this paper, the authors described how they arrived at the Minimum Alveolar Concentration (MAC) of anesthetic in the dog (Halothane) and in patients, which is necessary to prevent movement to a painful stimulus. The effective dose to anesthetize the spinal cord, MAC, was tested in various conditions including hemorrhage, hypocarbia, and hypercarbia with subsequent percent decrease in MAC. In another paper, authors Dr. Anis Barak and coworkers developed a Double T-Piece System for Rebreathing to be used for patients hyperventilating. *British Journal Anesthesiology*, 41 (1) (1969): 47–53. Doi:10.1093/brj/41.1.47.]
- (with E. I. Eger and L. Saidman) "Temperature Dependence of Halothane and Cyclopropane Anesthesia in Dogs; Correlation with Some Theories of Anesthetic Action," *Anesthesiology*, XXVI (1965): 764–770.
- (with E. I. Eger, L. Saidman, J. W. Severinghaus, and E. Munson) "Equipotent Alveolar Concentrations of Methoxyflurane, Halothane, Diethyl Ether, Fluroxene, Cyclopropane, Xenon and Nitrous Oxide in the Dog," *Anesthesiology*, XXVI (1965): 771–777.
- (with M. S. Slim, J. Bitar, S. Hajj, and H. G. Mishalani) "Congenital Anomalies: Etiology, Diagnosis and Surgical Considerations—Recent Advances in Pediatric Anesthesia," *Middle East Medical Journal*, II (1965): 24–42.

Kan'an, Munir A.

- (with H. G. Holek) "A Modified Class Demonstration of Difference between Ephedrine and Epinephrine Blood Pressure Response after Cocaine," *Proceedings of the Society for Experimental Biology and Medicine*, XXX (1933): 1087.
- (with H. G. Holek) "Intravenous Lethal Doses of Amytal in the Dog and Rabbit and a Table of Animal Dosages Compiled from the Literature," *Journal of Laboratory and Clinical Medicine*, XIX (1934): 1191–1205.
- (with H. G. Hokek) "Sex Difference in the White Rat in Tolerance to Certain Barbiturates," *Proceedings of the Society for Experimental Biology and Medicine*, XXXII (1935): 700–701. "Action of Morphine Sulfate on Intestinal Motility and Its Modification by Atropine Sulfate," *Proceedings of the Society for Experimental Biology and Medicine*, XXXVI (1937): 506.
- (with H. G. Holek, L. M. Mills, and E. L. Smith) "Studies upon the Sex Difference in Rats in Tolerance to Certain Barbiturates and to Nicotine," *Journal of Pharmacology and Experimental Therapy*, LX (1937): 1–24.
- "Drugs Used before and after Extraction of Teeth," *Lebanese Dental Magazine*, IV (1953): 41.
- "Dental Evidence in Forensic Medicine," *Lebanese Dental Magazine*, VII (1956): 27.

Muallem, Musa; chairman, 1969–1971

- The published contributions to anesthesiology of Dr. Muallem may be found online.
- The important basic science and clinical research published contributions of Dr. M. Muallem can be found or reseached under "Pub Med" and on the Internet.

Department of Bacteriology, Parasitology, and Virology

Berberian, Dikran

- (with H. A. Yenikomshian) "A Preliminary Report on the Incidence of Hookworm Disease in Syria and the Lebanon," *Transactions of the Royal Society of Tropical Medicine and Hygiene*, XXV (1932): 399–406.
- (with E. L. Turner and E. W. Dennis) "Successful Artificial Immunization of Dogs against Taenia Echinoccus," *Proceedings of the Society for Experimental Biology and Medicine*, XXX (1933): 618–619.
- (with E. W. Dennis) "Mechanism of Invasiveness in the Genus Streptococcus," *Proceedings of the Society for Experimental Biology and Medicine*, LX (1934): 581–598.
- (with E. W. Dennis) "A Study on the Mechanism of Invasiveness of Streptococci," *Journal of Experimental Medicine*, LX (1934): 581–598.

- (with E. W. Dennis) "A Study of the Production of Somatic and Flagellar Agglutinins in Response to Anti-Typhoid-Paratyphoid Inoculation," *American Journal of Hygiene*, XX (1934): 469–481.
- (with H. A. Yenikomshian) "The Occurrence and Distribution of Human Helminthiasis in Syria and the Lebanon," *Transactions of the Royal Society of Tropical Medicine and Hygiene*, XXVII (1934): 425–435.
- (with E. L. Turner and E. W. Dennis) "The Value of the Casoni Test in Dogs," *Journal of Parasitology*, XXI (1935): 180–182.
- (with E. L. Turner and E. W. Dennis) "The Production of Artificial Immunity in Dogs against Echinococcus Granulosus," *Journal of Parasitology*, XXII (1936): 14.
- "Some Observations on the Effect of Digestive Juices on Scolices of Echinococcus Granulosus (Batsch)," *Journal of Helminthology*, XIV (1936): 21–40.
- (with E. L. Turner and E. W. Dennis) "The Production of Artificial Immunity against Hydatid Disease in Sheep," *Journal of Parasitology*, XXIII (1937): 43–56.
- "A Method of Staining Hair and Epithelial Scales," *Archives of Dermatology and Syphilology*, XXXVI (1937): 1171–1175.
- "Successful Transmission of Cutaneous Leishmaniasis by the Bites of Stomoxys Calcitrans," *Proceedings of the Society for Experimental Biology and Medicine*, XXXVIII (1938): 254–256.
- "Dermatophytosis of the Feet, Sources and Methods of Prevention of Reinfection," *Archives of Dermatology and Syphilology*, XXXVIII (1938): 526–534.
- "Mycologic Technic for the Study of Anascosporous Yeast-like Fungi," *Archives of Dermatology and Syphilology*, XXXVIII (1938): 526–536.
- "Ringworm Infection of the Feet," *Journées Médicales de France et de l'Union Française*, II (1938).
- "Vaccination and Immunity against Oriental Sore," *Transactions of the Royal Society of Tropical Medicine and Hygiene*, XXXIII (1939): 87–94.
- "A Second Note on Successful Transmission of Oriental Sore on the Bites of Stomoxys Calcitrans," *Annals of Tropical Medicine and Parasitology*, XXXIII (1939): 95–96.
- "Interesting Cases of Tuberculosis of the Skin Stimulating Mycosis," *Urologic and Cutaneous Review*, XLV (1941): 317–320.
- "Studies on Cutaneous Leishmaniasis (Oriental Sore). I. Time Required for the Development of Immunity after Vaccination," *Archives of Dermatology and Syphilology*, XLIX (1944): 433–435.
- "Studies on Cutaneous Leishmaniasis (Oriental Sore). II. The Incubation Period of Oriental Sore," *Archives of Dermatology and Syphilology*, L (1944): 231–232.
- "Cutaneous Leishmaniasis (Oriental Sore). III. Period of Infectivity of Saline Suspensions of Leishmania tropica Cultures Kept at Room Temperature," *Archives of Dermatology and Syphilology*, L (1944): 233.

- "Cutaneous Leishmaniasis (Oriental Sore). IV. Vaccination against Oriental Sore with Suspensions of Killed Leishmania Tropica," *Archives of Dermatology and Syphilology*, L (1944): 234–236.
- "Cutaneous Leishmaniasis (Oriental Sore). V. Experimental Canine Cutaneous Leishmaniasis," *Archives of Dermatology and Syphilology*, LI (1945): 193–197.
- "Cutaneous Leishmaniasis (Oriental Sore). VI. Treatment with Quinacrine Hydrochloride," *Archives of Dermatology and Syphilology*, LII (1945): 26.
- "Etiology, Transmission and Prophylaxis of Dengue," *Revue Médicale du Moyen Orient*, IV (1945): 108.
- "Treatment of Lambiasis with Acranil," *American Journal of Tropical Medicine*, XXV (1945): 441–444.
- L'Empoisonment par le fromage en Syrie et au Liban, *Revue Médicale du Moyen Orient*, III (1945): 337–346.
- "Treatment of Hymenolepsis Nana Infection with Acranil," *American Journal of Tropical Medicine*, XXVI (1946): 339–343.
- "Cheese Poisoning in Syria and Lebanon," *Journal of the Palestine Arab Medical Association*, I (1946): 30.
- "The Species of Anopheline Mosquitos Found in Syria and Lebanon, Their Habits, Distribution and Eradication," *Journal of the Palistine Arab Medical Association*, I (July 1946): 120–146.
- (with E. W. Dennis) "Field Experiments with Chloroquine Diphosphate," *American Journal of Tropical Medicine*, XXVIII (1948): 755–776.
- "Host Specificity and the Effect of Digestive Juices on Ova of Echinococcus Granulosus," *Annual Report of the Oriental Hospital*, X (1957): 33–43.
- (with R. J. Pauly and M. L. Tainter) "Comparison of a Plain Methyl-Cellulose with a Compound Bulk Laxative Tablet," *Gastroenterology*, XX (1952): 43–48.
- (with E. W. Dennis) "Tropical Diseases," *Annual Review of Medicine*, IV (1953): 345–372.
- (with H. O. Paquin Jr., and A. Fantauzzi) "Longevity of Schistosoma Hematobium and Schistosoma Mansoni: Observations Based on Case," *Journal of Parasitology*, XXXIX (1953): 517–519.
- (with E. W. Dennis) "Chemotherapeutic Properties of Win 5047 (Mantomide) New Synthetic Amebacide," *Antibiotics and Chemotherapy*, IV (1954): 554–560.
- "Trichomonacidal Activity of Milibis (Glycobiarsol)," *New York Medical Journal*, LIV (1954): 3102–3105.
- "Treatment of Ménière's Disease with Apolamine," *American Practitioner and Digest of Treatment*, VII (1956): 1425–1428.
- (with E. Rizk and E. W. Dennis) "Mass Suppression of Hyperendemic Vivax Malaria with Hydroxychloroquine," *Lebanese Medical Journal*, XIII (1960): 54–70.
- (with R. G. Slighter and E. W. Dennis) "N, N'–Bis (dichloroacetyl) Diamines as Amebicidal Agents," *American Journal of Tropical Medicine and Hygiene*, X (1961): 503.

- (with A. Arnold and S. D. Sobell) "Maintenance of Elevated Blood Levels of Vitamin (B12) in Human Subjects," *American Journal of Clinical Nutrition*, X (1962): 56–58.

Djanian, Aida

- (with W. M. Shanklin and J. M. Butros) "Effect of Tubercle Bacilli Extracts on Induced Tumors of the Rat," *Cancer Research*, IX (1949): 520–525.
- (with C. Nassar and W. M. Shanklin) "The Etiological Significance of Ergot in the Incidence of Post-Partum Necrosis of the Anterior Pituitary. A Preliminary Report," *American Journal of Obstetrics and Gynecology*, LX (1950): 140–145.
- "VDRL Tube Test. A Comparison with the Kahn and Kolmer Tests for Syphilis," *British Journal of Venereal Diseases*, XXIX (1953): 238–239.
- (with G. A. Garabedian and E. A. Johnston) "Q Fever in Lebanon (Middle East). I. The Presence of Complement—Fixing Antibodies in Serum Samples Obtained from Residents of Lebanon," *American Journal of Hygiene*, LXIII (1956): 308–312.
- (with G. A. Garabedian) "Q Fever in Lebanon (Middle East). II. Attempts to Demonstrate by Animal Inoculation the Presence of C. *burneti* in Milk Samples," *American Journal of Hygiene*, LXIII (1956): 313–318.
- (with G. A. Garabedian and R. M. Matossian) "An Indirect Hemagglutination Test for Hydatid Disease," *Journal of Immunology*, LXXVIII (1957): 269–272.
- (with G. A. Garabedian and R. M. Matossian) "Serologic Diagnosis of Hydatid Disease by Indirect Hemagglutination," *Lebanese Medical Journal*, X (1957): 275–282.

Garabedian, Garabed A.; chairman of the Department of Bacteriology (Microbiology), Parasitology, and Virology

- (with J. E. Azar and A. C. Pipkin) "An Intensive Treatment Regimen of Vesical Schistosomiasis with Fuadin," *American Journal of Tropical Medicine*, XXIX (1949): 595–604.
- (with E. Rizk, H. T. Chaglassian, and A. C. Pipkin) "Studies on Treponemes of Bejal—Part I. History, Morphologic Characteristics and Staining Properties," *American Journal of Syphilis, Gonorrhea and Venereal Diseases*, XXXV (1951): 201–206.
- (with E. Rizk and E. I. Shwayri) "Studies on the Treponemes of Bejal—Part II. Transmission to Rabbits and Observation on the Course of Experimental Infection," *American Journal of Syphilis, Gonorrhea and Venereal Diseases*, XXXV (1951): 207–215.
- (with A. Donabedian and F. Abu Haidar) "Studies on a Recent Epidemic of Influenza—A Preliminary Report," *Lebanese Medical Journal*, VII (1954): 146–154.
- (with J. T. Syverton) "Studies on Herpes Simplex Virus. I. An Antigenic Analysis of Four Strains of Virus Isolated from a Human Subject," *Journal of Infectious Diseases*, XCVI (1955): 1–4.

- (with J. T. Syverton) "Studies on Herpes Simplex Virus. II. An Affinity *on vitro* of Herpes Virus for Rabbit Microphages and Macrophages," *Journal of Infectious Diseases*, XCVI (1955): 5–8.
- (with J. T. Syverton and J. Friedman) "Studies on Herpes Simplex Virus. III. The Effects of Roentgen Radiation, Cortizone and Gastric Mucin upon the Infectivity of Herpes Simplex Virus for Laboratory Mice," *Journal of Infectious Diseases*, XCVI (1955): 9–13.
- (with A. Donabedian and F. Abu Haidar) "Studies on an Outbreak of Influenza in Beirut, Lebanon," *American Journal of Tropical Medicine and Hygiene*, V (1956): 642–646.
- (with A. Y. Djanian and E. A. Johnston) "Q Fever in Lebanon (Middle East). I. The Presence of Complement—Fixing Antibodies in Serum Samples Obtained from Residents of Lebanon," *American Journal of Hygiene*, LXIII (1956): 308–312.
- (with A. Y. Djanian) "Q Fever in Lebanon (Middle East). II. Attempts to Demonstrate by Animal Inoculation the Presence of C. *burneti* in Milk Samples," *American Journal of Hygiene*, LXIII (1956): 313–318.
- (with R. M. Matossian and A. Y. Djanian) "An Indirect Hemagglutination Test for Hydatid Disease," *Journal of Immunology*, LXXVIII (1957): 269–272.
- (with R. M. Matossian and A. Y. Djanian) "Serologic Diagnosis of Hydatid Disease by Indirect Hemagglutination," *Lebanese Medical Journal*, X (1957): 275–282.
- (with R. M. Matossian and F. G. Suidan) "A Correlative Study of Immunological Tests for the Diagnosis of Hydatid Disease," *American Journal of Tropical Medicine and Hygiene*, VIII (1959): 67–71.
- (with A. H. Malakian and R. M. Matossian) "A Simple Hemagglutination Drop Test for Human Hydatidosis," *Annals of Tropical Medicine and Parasitology*, LIV (1960): 233–235.
- (with J. T. Syverton) "Detection of Anti-He La Antibodies in Rabbit Antiserum by Indirect Hemagglutination," *Proceedings of the Society for Experimental Biology and Medicine*, CV (1960): 632–635.
- (with R. M. Matossian and A. H. Malakian) "Status of Typhus in Lebanon," *American Journal of Tropical Medicine and Hygiene*, XI (1962): 104–107.
- (with R. M. Matossian and J. Thaddeus) "Outbreak of Epidemic Typhus in the Northern Region of Saudi Arabia," *American Journal of Tropical Medicine and Hygiene*, XII (1963): 82–90.
- (with R. M. Matossian and J. Hatem) "Poliomyelitis in Lebanon. A Statistical, Serological and Virological Study," *Lebanese Medical Journal*, XVI (1963): 216–229.
- (with R. M. Matossian, N. Balassamian and J. Hatem) "La Poliomylite paralytique au Liban en 1962," *Revue Médicale du Moyen Orient*, XXI (1964) : 25–31. [**Nassar comment:** Recent attention has alerted clinicians to the entity of post-polio syndrome, which develops many years following paralytic polio and is probably not related to a resurgent dormant polio virus type 1, 2, or 3. It is thought to be due to poor recovery of the paralyzed limb muscles. Reference: D. A. Trojan and N. R. Cashman,

"Post-Polio Syndrome, Muscle Nerve," 31 (1) 2005, 6-19; "Post-Polio Syndrome Fact Sheet," National Institute of Nervous Disorders and Stroke 2011.]

- (with R. M. Matossian and J. Hatem) "Les Rickettsioses au Liban," *Review de Pathologie Comparée et d'Hygiène Général,* LXIV (1964): 533–536.
- (with J. Hatem and R. M. Matossian) "L'évolution de la Poliomyélite au Liban au Cours de l'après-gurre," *Gazette des Hôpitaux Civils et Militaires,* CXXXVI (1964): 1337–1340.
- "The Behavior of Tanned Erythrocytes in Various Hemagglutination Systems," *Journal of General Microbiology,* XXXVIII (1965): 181–187.
- (with R. M. Matossian and J. Hatem) "Current Status of Bacterial, Rickettsial and Viral Infections in Lebanon," *Lebanese Medical Journal,* XVIII (1965): 103–125.

Hatem, Joseph M. (published book manuals and papers on infectious diseases)

- *Standard Laboratory Methods in Microbiology.* Beirut: Central public health laboratory, Ministry of Health, 1959.
- (with R. M. Matossian) *Laboratory Instructions in Bacteriology for Laboratory Technicians.* Beirut: American University of Beirut, 1964.
- La poliomyelite au Liban et leur interpretation. *Rev. Med. Moy.Or.,* XVII (1960): 9–17.
- (with J. Chidiac) Title translated from French: "An Inquiry into a Case of Recurrent Fever," *Rev. Med. Moy. Or.,* XVII (1960): 504–505.
- (with E. Stephan) A Propos d'un cas de Typhus murin. *Rev. Med. Moy. Or.,* XVII (1960): 505–507.
- "Investigation of a Case of Poliomyelitis Occurring during Polio Vaccination," *Lebanese Medical Journal,* XIII (1960): 600–802.
- Contribution du Laboratoire au control sanitaire des produits laitiers au Liban. *Rev. Med. Moy. Or.,* XVII (1960): 453–460.
- Intoxication collective par la creme glace'e. *Rev. Med. Moy. Or.,* XVII (1960): 600–602.
- La rube'ole maternelle, facteur teratogene. *J. Med. Lib.,* XVI (1960): 234–237.
- Comment concilier les exigencies de la therapeutique modernes et les lemteurs du laboratoire Dans le diagnostic des salmonelloses. *Rev. Med. Moy. Or.,* XVIII (1961): 61–83.
- (with A. Ghossain) Un nouveau cas de Charbom intestinal. *Rev. Med. Moy. Or.,* XVIII (1961): 505–506.
- (with A. Merab, N. Taleb, and W. Nasr) Le Toxi-Infections alimentaires au Liban. *Press Med.* LXIX (1961): 2132–2134.
- (with A. Ghossain) Le Charbon intestinal, *Press Med.* LXXI (1963): 1059–1062.
- (with G. A. Garabedian and R. M. Matossian) "Poliomyelitis in Lebanon: A Statistical, Serological, and Virological study," *Lebanese Medical Journal,* XVI (1963): 216–229.
- (with R. M. Matossian, G. A. Garabedian, and N. Balassanian) "Paralytic Poliomyelitis in Lebanon in 1962," *Rev. Med. Myo. Or.,* XXI "1964": 25–34 (translated from French).

- (with R. M. Matossian, and G. A. Garbedian) "The Evolution of Poliomyelitis in Lebanon in Its Course after the War," *Gazette des Hôpitaux Civils et Militaires*, CXXXVI (1964): 1337–1340 (translated from French).
- (with R. M. Matossian and G. A. Garabedian) "Rickettsioses in Lebanon," (title translated from French). *Review de Pathologie Comparée et d'Hygiène Général*, LXIV (1964): 533–536.
- (with R. M. Matossian, and G. A. Garabedian) "Current Status of Bacterial, Rikettsial, and Viral Infections in Lebanon," *Lebanese Medical Journal*, XVIII (1965): 103–125.

Mayer, Edmund

- "Tissue Culture Colonies In-Vitro," *Tabulae Biologicae*, XIX (1939).[38]

Rizk, Emile

- (with H. T. Chaglassian, G. A. Garabedian, and A. C. Pipkin) "Studies on Treponemes of Bejel—Part I. History, Morphologic Characteristics and Staining Properties," *American Journal of Syphilis, Gonorrhea and Venereal Diseases*, XXXV (1951): 201–206.
- (with G. A. Garabedian and E. I. Shwayri) "Studies on the Treponemes of Bejel—Part II. Transmission to Rabbits and Observation on the Course of Experimental Infection," *American Journal of Syphilis, Gonorrhea and Venereal Diseases*, XXXV (1951): 207–215.
- (with H. Zellweger and M. Salam) "Intestinal Parasitism in Lebanon," *Ann. Paediat.* (Basel), CLXXXV (1955): 310–319.

Schwabe, Calvin W.; chairman of Department of Parasitology, 1956–1966 (papers on infectious disease and parasitology)

- *Veterinary Medicine and Human Health* (Baltimore: Williams and Wilkins Co., 1864), 516.
- (with K. A. Daoud) "A Skin Test for Histoplasmosis and Coccidioidiomycosis in the Middle East," *Am. Journal of Tropical Medicine and Hygiene*, VII (1958): 643.
- "What Is Halzoun," *Lebanese Medical Journal*, XI (1958): 42–44.
- "Notes on Ancient Egyptian Veterinary Practices," *Auburn Veterinarian*, XV (1958): 1–8.
- "Host-Parasite Relationships in Echinococcosis. I. Observations on the Permeability of the Hydatid Cyst Wall," *Am. Journal of Tropical Medicine and Hygiene*, VIII (1959): 20–28.

---

38 This paper is ahead of its time. It has been only within the past four to five decades that tissue culture has become exceedingly important.

- (with I. Farhan and C. R. Zebel) "Host-Parasite Relationships in Echinococcosis. III. Relation of Environmental Oxygen Tension to the Metabolism of the Scolices," *Am. Journal of Tropical Medicine and Hygiene*, VIII (1959): 474–477.

- (with M. Koussa, and N. N. Acra) "Host-Parasite Relationships in Echinococcosis. IV. Acetylcholine-Esterase and Permeability in the Hydatid Cyst Wall," *Comparative Biochemistry and Physiology II* (1960): 161–172.

- (with E. Meymerian) "Host-Parasitic Relationships in Echinococcosis. VII. Resistance of Ova of Echinococcus Granulose to Germicide," *Am. J. Trop. Hyg.*, XI (1962): 360.

Department of Biochemistry

Al-Khalidi, Usama A. S.

- (editor with I. F. Durr, A. K. Khachadurian, and J. G. Reinhold) *Selected Papers in Biochemistry and Related Topics* (Beirut, 1965).

- (with S. E. Kerr) "Molecular Size and Branching of Ribonucleic Acid," *Proceedings of the Third International Congress of Biochemistry* (1955): 23.

- (with G. I. Abu Haydar, F. Chernijoy, and S. E. Kerr) "A Titrimetric Method for the Determination of the Molecular Weight of Small Polynucleotides," *Journal of Biological Chemistry*, CCXXVIII (1957): 487–493.

- "Riboflavin Biosynthesis," *Federation Proceedings*, XVII (1958): 180.

- "Unidentified Guanine Metabolite Formed by Extracts of *E. ashbyii*," *Federation Proceedings* XVIII (1959): 180.

- (with G. R. Guenberg) "Isolation of 2 (α–Propionamino)–6–Hydroxypurine (Guanine Propionate)," *Journal of Biological Chemistry*, CCXXXVI (1961): 189–191.

- (with G. R. Guenberg) "The Structure of Guanine Propionate," *Journal of Biological Chemistry*, CCXXXVI (1961): 192–196.

- (with A. K. Khachadurian) "Biochemistry of Cancer," *Journal of the Iraqi Medical Society*, IX (1961): 1–5.

- "The Synthesis of Guanine Propionate through the Leukart Reaction," *Proceedings of the Fifth International Conference of Biochemistry*, (1961): 1.

- (with M. H. Shamma'a) "Dietary Carbohydrates and Serum Cholesterol in Man," *American Journal of Clinical Nutrition*, XIII (1963): 194–196.

- (with S. Nasrallah) "Nature of Purines Excreted in Urine during Muscular Exercise," *Journal of Applied Physiology*, XIX (1964): 246–248.

- (with M. H. Shamma'a) "Uptake of Cholesterol by Segments of Small Intestine of Rat," *American Journal of Physiology*, CCVII (1964): 33–36. [**Nassar comment:** Also referenced with Dr. Munir H. Shamma'a being the first author. These experiments on radioactive labeled cholesterol absorption in small intestinal segments of the small intestine of rat are an attempt to delineate the mechanisms involved in cholesterol migration from the lumen to the serosal surface and the lympatics. In the rat, cholesterol is not absorbed in the large intestine; second, aside from problem of cholesterol absorption, there appears to be a small portion of cholesterol absorbed passively, and for its appearance in the serosal surface takes about two to three days reported by few investigators *in vivo* experiments. However, the authors suggest a gradient being involved for cholesterol absorption; moreover, absorption from the intestinal small segment is decreased in the presence of acidic bile. In conclusion, several mechanisms are involved in small intestinal cholesterol absorption with an energy gradient involved even though there is no high temperature coeffient noted.]

- (with A. K. Khachadurian, S. Nasrallah, and M. H. Shamma'a) "A Sensitive Method for Determination of Xanthine Oxidase Activity," *Clinical Chemistry Acta*, XI (1965): 72–77. [**Nassar comment:** The authors describe a radioactive sensitive method for the determination of xanthine oxidase activity demonstrating a much more accurate method than the standard assays reported in the literature. The clinical significance is that such a sensitive assay of xanthine oxidase that catalyzes hypoxanthine and xanthine for the metabolic product of uric acid in the serum or blood will improve the diagnosis of hyperuricemia or not in samples of serum or blood.]

- (with M. H. Shamma'a) "Serum Xanthine Oxidase Determination and Hepatic Disease," *Lebanese Medical Journal*, XVII (1964): 231–232. [**Nassar comment:** The author discusses the usefulness of measuring the enzyme xanthine oxidase in liver injury or inflammation. The enzyme activity is specific in the liver and small intestine, though it does not carry any prognostic significance. In a comparative analysis, the enzyme was markedly elevated in viral hepatitis but not so in obstructive jaundice.]

- (with M. H. Shamma'a, S. Nasrallah, T. Chaglassian, and A. K. Khachadurian) "Serum Xanthine Oxidase, a Sensitive Test of Acute Liver Injury," *Gastroenterology*, XLVIII (1965): 226–230.

- (with T. Chaglassian) "The Species Distribution of Xanthine Oxidase," *Biochemical Journal*, (in press).

- (with M. H. Shamma'a and S. Nasrallah) "Serum Xanthine Oxidase in Differential Diagnosis of Jaundice," *Journal of Laboratory and Clinical Medicine*, (in press).

- (with M. H. Shamma'a and R. Jeha) "The Comparative Sensitivity of Serum Xanthine Oxidase, Glutamic Oxalometic and Glutamic Pyrudic Transaminases in Carbon Tetrachloride Induced Hepatic Necrosis in Sheep," *Biochimica et Biophysica Acta*, (in press).

- (with M. H. Shamma'a and S. Hajj) "Serum Xanthine Oxidase in Obstetrical Conditions," *American Journal of Obstetrics and Gynecology*, (in press).

Avery, Bennett F.

- (with A. B. Hastings) "A Gasometric Method for the Determination of Lactic Acid in the Blood," *Journal of Biological Chemistry*, XCIV (1931): 273–280.

- (with L. W. Parr) "The Relation of the Dick Test to the Prevalence of Scarlet Fever in Grand Lebanon," *J. Prevent. Med.*, I (1927): 529–536.
- (with A. K. Mufarrij) "Ultraviolet Irradiation of the Blood Stream in Septicemia," *Proceedings of the Society for Experimental Biology and Medicine*, XL (1939): 436–438.

Blish, Mary

- (with S. E. Kerr) "The Effect of Insulin on the Distribution of Phosphorus in Muscle," *Journal of Biological Chemistry*, XCVII (1932): 11–22.
- (with S. E. Kerr) "A Method for the Determination of Nucleotide in Blood and Muscle," *Journal of Biological Chemistry*, XCVIII (1932): 103–205.
- (with A. Bodansky and P. F. Sahyoun) "Experimental Fetal Nephritis," *Proceedings of the Society for Experimental Biology and Medicine*, XXXI (1933): 7–13.

Durr, Ibrahim F.

- (editor with A. K. Khachadurian, U. A. S. al-Khalidi, and J. G. Reinhold) *Selected Papers in Biochemistry and Related Topics*, (Beirut, 1965).
- "Structure-Activity Relationships among the Steroids," *Lebanese Pharmaceutical Journal*, VI (1960): 57–80.
- "The Hydrolysis of (2-Acetylmercaptoethyl) Trimethylammonium Iodide in Yeast," *Journal of Biological Chemistry*, CCXXXVIII (1963): 728–733.
- "The Biochemical Approach to the Study of Disease and Therapy," *Lebanese Pharmaceutical Journal*, VIII (1963): 65–81.
- (with N. Cortas) "The Reduction of Pantethine by an Extract of Camel Intestine," *Biochemical Journal*, XCI (1964): 460–463.
- (with A. Shwaryi) "The Metabolism of Mevalonic Acid by Lactobacillus Plantarum," *Journal of Bacteriology*, LXXXVIII (1964): 361–366.
- (with B. Dajani) "Oxidative Pathways in the Adipose Tissue of the Fat-Tail Sheep," *Comparative Biochemistry and Physiology*, XIII (1964): 225–232.

Kerr, Stanley E.; professor emeritus and chairman of the Department of Biochemistry

- "Studies on the Inorganic Composition of Blood. I. The Effect of Hemorrhage on the Inorganic Composition of Serum and Corpuscles," *Journal of Biological Chemistry*, LXVII (1926): 689–720.
- "Studies on the Inorganic Composition of Blood. II. Changes in the Potassium Content of Erythrocytes under Certain Experimental Conditions," *Journal of Biological Chemistry*, LXVII (1926): 721–735.
- "The Effect of Insulin and Pancreatectomy on the Distribution of Phosphorous and Potassium in the Blood," *Journal of Biological Chemistry*, LXXVIII (1928): 35–52.

[**Nassar comment:** Two experiments were designed: (1) A study of the effect of insulin overdosage on the distribution of inorganic phosphorous, acid soluble phosphorous, lipid phosphorous and potassium between the serum and red blood corpuscles. Results: the content of corpuscles was not significantly increased and that the effect on organic phosphorous, insulin does not cause a synthesis of phosphoric estersin in the red blood corpuscles in dogs. (2) The effect of insulin overdosage in pancreatectomised dogs on organic phosphorous and blood potassium. Result: The potassium serum level disappears but does not enter the corpuscles.]

- (with V. Krikorian) "The Effect of Insulin on the Distribution of Non-Protein Nitrogen in the Blood," *Journal of Biological Chemistry*, LXXXI (1929): 421–424.
- "Studies on the Inorganic Composition of Blood. III. The Influence of Serum on the Permeability of Erythrocytes to Potassium and Sodium," *Journal of Biological Chemistry*, LXXXV (1930): 47–64.
- (with M. E. Blish) "The Effect of Insulin on the Distribution of Phosphorous in Muscle," *Journal of Biological Chemistry*, XCVII (1932): 11–22. [**Nassar comment:** The experiment included the study of phosphocreatine content in cardiac muscle of rabbits. The results have clinical implications in human cardiac muscle because phosphocreatine is an energy source involved in the reduction of adenotriphosphate to adenodiphosphate (ATP$\longleftrightarrow$ADP) and its restoration to ATP. This is of importance in understanding energy sources of cardiac contraction in normal human hearts and in congestive heart failure.]
- (with M. E. Blish) "A Method for the Determination of Nucleotides in Blood and Muscle," *Journal of Biological Chemistry*, XCVIII (1932): 193–205.
- (with L. Daoud) "A Study of the Organic Acid-Soluble Phosphorous of the Erythrocytes of Various Vertebrates," *Journal of Biological Chemistry*, CIX (1935): 301–315.
- "Studies on the Phosphorous Compounds of Brain. I. Phosphocreatine," *Journal of Biological Chemistry*, CX (1935): 625–635.
- (with B. F. Avery and M. Ghantus) "The Lactic Acid Compound of Mammalian Brain," *Journal of Biological Chemistry*, CX (1935): 637–642.
- "The Carbohydrate Metabolism of Brain. I. Glycogen," *Journal of Biological Chemistry*, CXVI (1936): 1–7. [**Nassar comment:** The astute Dr. Kerr noted the errors in various reported results in biochemical literature when glycogen was determined in tissues using the Pfluger method, which resulted in wide variety of values for glycogen (0–269 mg per 100 gm). With careful modifications to eliminate errors in the method, Dr. Kerr was able to determine the glycogen of brain in the dog (seven experiments), in the cat (five experiments), in the rabbit (five experiments), and in the sea turtle (four experiments). By such modified methods, the percent recovery of glycogen in the mammalian brain averaged 95.6 percent, or 70–130 mg per 100 gm of brain frozen *in situ*.]
- (with M. Ghantus) "The Carbohydrate Metabolism of Brain. II. The Effect of Varying the Carbohydrate and Insulin Supply on the Glycogen, Free Sugar and Lactic Acid in Mammalian Brain," *Journal of Biological Chemistry*, CXVI (1936): 9–20.

- (with M. Ghantus) "The Carbohydrate Metabolism of Brain. III. On the Origin of Lactic Acid," *Journal of Biological Chemistry*, CXVII (1937): 217–225.
- "Studies on the Inorganic Composition of Blood. IV. The Relationship of Potassium to the Acid-Soluble Phosphorous Fractions," *Journal of Biological Chemistry*, CXVII (1937): 227–235.
- (with C. W. Hampel and M. Ghantus) "The Carbohydrate Metabolism of Brain. IV. Brain Glycogen, Free Sugar and Lactic Acid as Affected by Insulin in Normal and Adrenal-Inactivated Cats, and by Epinephrine in Normal Rabbits," *Journal of Biological Chemistry*, CXVIII (1937): 405–421.
- (with A. Antaki) "On the Nature of the Organic Phosphorous of Blood Hydrolyzed by the Phosphatases of Bone, Kidney and Blood," *Journal of Biological Chemistry*, CXIX (1937): 531.
- (with A. Antaki) "The Carbohydrate Metabolism of Brain. V. The Effect of Certain Narcotics and Convulsant Drugs upon the Carbohydrate and Phosphocreatine Content of Rabbit Brain," *Journal of Biological Chemistry*, CXXII (1937): 49–52.
- "Note on the Phosphorous Content of Rat Brain in Experimental Rickets," *Journal of Biological Chemistry*, CXXII (1937): 53–54.
- "The Carbohydrate Metabolism of Brain. VI. Isolation of Glycogen," *Journal of Biological Chemistry*, CXXIII (1938): 443–449.
- (with K. Seraidarian) "The Determination of Purine Nucleotides and Nucleosides in Blood and Tissues," *Journal of Biological Chemistry*, CXXXII (1940): 147–159.
- (with K. Seraidarian) "On the Preparation of Adenosine Triphosphate," *Journal of Biological Chemistry*, CXXXIX (1941): 121–130.
- "Notes on the Preparation of Muscle Adenylic Acid," *Journal of Biological Chemistry*, CXXXIX (1941): 131–134.
- (with K. Seraidarian) "Studies on the Phosphorous Compounds of Brain. II. Adenosine Triphosphate," *Journal of Biological Chemistry*, CXL (1941): 77–81.
- (with R. J. Pauly) "Invert Sugar as a Substitute for Glucose in Intravenous Therapy," *Surgery, Gynecology and Obstetrics with International Abstracts of Surgery*, LXXIV (1942): 925–927.
- (with K. Seraidarian) "Studies on the Phosphorous Compounds of Brain. III. Determinations of Adenosine Triphosphate and Its Decomposition Products in Fresh and Autolyzed Dog Brain," *Journal of Biological Chemistry*, CXLV (1942): 647–656.
- (with K. Seraidarian) "The Separation of Purine Nucleosides from Free Purines and the Determination of the Purines and Ribose in these Fractions," *Journal of Biological Chemistry*, CLIX (1945): 211–225.
- (with K. Seraidarian) "The Pathway of Decomposition of Myoadenylic Acid during Autolysis in Various Tissues," *Journal of Biological Chemistry*, CLIX (1945): 637–645.
- (with M. Wargon and K. Seraidarian) "On the Composition of Pancreas Ribonucleic Acid," *Proceedings of the First International Congress of Biochemistry*, (1949): 625–627.

- (with K. Seraidarian) "Studies on Ribonucleic Acid. I. Preparation from Pancreas," *Journal of Biological Chemistry*, CLXXX (1949): 1203–1208.
- (with M. Wargon and K. Seraidarian) "Studies on Ribonucleic Acid. II. Methods of Analysis," *Journal of Biological Chemistry*, CLXXXI (1949): 761–771.
- (with M. Wargon and K. Seraidarian) "Studies on Ribonucleic Acid. III. Composition of Pancreas Ribonucleic Acid," *Journal of Biological Chemistry*, CLXXXI (1949): 773–780.
- (with K. Seraidarian and G. B. Brown) "On the Utilization of Purines and Their Ribose Derivatives by Yeast," *Journal of Biological Chemistry*, CLXXXVIII (1951): 207–216.
- (with L. Cavalieri and A. Angelos) "On the Structure of Ribonucleic Acid," *Journal of the American Chemistry Society*, LXXIII (1951): 2567–2578.
- (with F. Chernijoy) "On the Biosynthesis of Ribonucleic Acid Purines and Their Interconversion in Yeast," *Journal of Biological Chemistry*, CC (1953): 887–894.
- (with N. Waked) "The Distribution of Phosphomonoesterases and Pyrophosphatase in the Particulate Fractions of Dog Cerebrum," *Journal of Histochemistry and Cytochemistry*, III (1955): 75–84.
- (with U. A. S. al-Khalidi) "Molecular Size and Branching of Ribonucleic Acid," *Proceedings of the Third International Congress of Biochemistry*, (1955): 23.
- (with G. I. Abu Haydar, F. Chernijoy, and A. K. Khachadurian) "Incorporation of C14 Labelled Glycine and Formate by the Acid-Soluble Guanine and Adenine Nucleotides of Rat Liver," *Journal of Biological Chemistry*, CCXXIV (1957): 707–712.
- (with U. A. S. al-Khalidi, G. I. Abu Haydar, and F. Chernijoy) "A Titrimetric Method for the Determination of the Molecular Weight of Small Polynucleotides," *Journal of Biological Chemistry*, CCXXVIII (1957): 487–493.
- (with F. Chernijoy) "Note on the Preparation of Prostate Phosphomonoesterase Free from Ribonuclease," *Journal of Biological Chemistry*, CCXXVIII (1957): 495–497.
- (with G. A. Kfoury) "Chromatographic Separation and Identification of Myoinositol Phosphates," *Archives of Biochemistry and Biophysics*, XCVI (1962): 347–353.
- (with G. A. Kfoury and L. G. Djibelian) "On the Nature of Dialyzable Phosphate Associated with the Di- and Tri-Phosphoinositides of Brain Phospholopids," *Biochimica et Biophysica Acta*, LXX (1963): 474–476.
- (with U. A. S. al-Khalidi) "Metabolism of Adipose Tissue in the Fat Tail Sheep," *Federation Proceedings*, XXII (1963): 471.
- (with W. W. C. Read) "The Fatty Acid Components of Polyphosphoinositide Prepared from Calf Brain," *Biochimica et Biophysica Acta*, LXX (1963): 477–478.
- (with G. A. Kfoury and L. G. Djibelian) "Preparation of Brain Polyphosphoinositides," *Journal of Lipid Research*, V (1964): 481–483.
- (with G. A. Kfoury) "On the Occurrence of Diphosphoinositol in the Lipids of Liver and Pancreas," *Biochimica et Biophysica Acta*, LXXXIV (1964): 391–403.
- (with G. A. Kfoury and F. S. Haddad) "A Comparison of the Polyphosphoinositide in Human and Ox Brain," *Biochimica et Biophysica Acta*, LXXXIV (1963): 461–463.

Khachadurian, Avedis K.; professor of biochemistry and internal medicine

- (editor with U. A. S. al-Khalidi, I. F. Durr, and J. G. Reinhold) *Selected Papers in Biochemistry and Related Papers* (Beirut, 1965).
- (with H. S. Badeer) "Effect of Hypothermia on Oxygen Consumption and Energy Utilization of Heart," *Circulation Research*, IV (1956): 523–526.
- (with G. I. Abu Haydar, F. Chernijoy, and S. E. Kerr) "Incorporation of C14 Labelled Glycine and Formate by the Acid-Soluble Guanine and Adenine Nucleotides of Rat Liver," *Journal of Biological Chemistry*, CCXXIV (1957): 707–712.
- (with H. S. Badeer) "Role of Bradycardia and Cold Per Se in Increasing Mechanical Efficiency of Hypothermic Heart," *American Journal of Physiology*, CXCII (1958): 331–334.
- (with K. Abu Feisal) "Alkaptonuria: Report of a Family with Seven Cases Appearing in Four Successive Generations, with Metabolic Studies in One Patient," *Journal of Chronic Diseases*, VII (1958): 455–465.
- (with R. C. DeMeutter and A. Marble) "Immediate Effects of Intravenous Injections of Tolbutamide and Insulin on Blood Glucose and Amino Acids," *Proceedings of the Society for Experimental Biology and Medicine*, XCIX (1958): 33–35.
- (with W. H. Hadley and A. Marble) "Studies with Chlorpropamide in Diabetic Patients," *Annals of the New York Academy of Sciences*, LXXIV (1959): 621–624.
- (with W. E. Knox and A. Cullen) "Colorimetric Ninhydrin Method for Total Alpha Amino Acids of Urine," *Journal of Laboratory and Clinical Medicine*, LVI (1960): 321–332.
- (with H. S. Badeer) "Effect of Tolbutamide on Glucose Utilization by Denervated Heart-Lung Preparation," *Metabolism*, IX (1960): 890–896.
- (with J. D. Karam and H. S. Badeer) "Effect of Tolbutamide on Glucose and Oxygen Uptake and Coronary Flow in the Isolated Dog Heart," *Arch. Int. Pharmacodyn.*, CXXXII (1961): 42–48.
- (with U. A. S. al-Khalidi) "Biochemistry of Cancer," *Journal of the Iraqi Medical Society*, IX (1961): 1–5.
- "Amino-Aciduria Secondary to a Functioning Parathyroid Carcinoma," *Annals of Internal Medicine*, LVI (1962): 931–934.
- "Essential Hyperlipemia," *Middle East Medical Journal*, I (1962): 13–24.
- "Essential Pentosuria," *American Journal of Human Genetics*, XIV (1962): 249–255.
- (with S. E. Kerr) "The Metabolism of Adipose Tissue in the Fat Tail Sheep," *Federation Proceedings*, XXII (1963): 471.
- "Nonalimentary Fructosuria," *Pediatrics*, XXXII (1963): 455–457.
- "The Inheritance of Essential Familial Hypercholesterolemia," *American Journal of Medicine*, XXXVII (1964): 402–407.
- (with L. A. Khachadurian) "The Inheritance of Renal Glycosuria," *American Journal of Human Genetics*, XVI (1964): 189.

- (with U. A. S. al-Khalidi, S. Nasrallah, and M. H. Shamma'a) "A Sensitive Method for the Determination of Xanthine Oxidase Activity," *Clinica Chimica Acta*, VII (1964): 72–77.
- (with M. Shamma'a, S. Nasrallah, T. Chaglassian, and U. A. S. al-Khalidi) "Serum Xanthine Oxidase. A Sensitive Test of Acute Liver Injury," *Gastroenterology*, XLVIII (1965): 226– 230.
- (with A. F. Obeid) "Nephropathy Secondary to Essential Familial Hyperlipemia," *Lebanese Medical Journal*, XVII (1964): 413–419.
- (with A. F. Obeid) "Nephropathy in Essential Familial Hyperlipaemia," *Lancet*, II (1964): 911–912.
- (with I. Somerville) "Diabetes Mellitus in Lebanon. A Retrospective Clinical Study of 560 Patients," *Journal of Chronic Diseases*, XVIII (1965): 1309–1315.
- (with B. Adrouni and H. D. Yacoubian) "Metabolism of Adipose Tissue in the Fat Tail of the Sheep *in vivo*," *Journal of Lipid Research*, VII (1966): 427–436.

Khairallah, Philip

- "Nucleotide Metabolism in Cardiac Activity," *Nature*, CLXXXIII (1959): 181. [**Nassar comment:** Dr. Khairallah and Dr. W. R. H. M. Mommaerts in a subsequent publication: "Nucleotide Metabolism in Cardiac Activity II: Reactions in Systole," *Circ. Research* (1953), studied the nucleotide content of the resting myocardium and the breakdown of adenosine triphosphate (ATP) in one single contraction, i.e., systole. When they compared the content of nucleotide (ATP) in relaxed myocardium to contraction activity, systole, the content of ATP was reduced to one-tenth in value and that ATP was dephosphorylated to adenosine diphosphate (ADP). The importance of this investigative preclinical scientific research supports the work of Dr. G. A. Fawaz and his synthesis of phosphocreatine which is involved in providing energy to the reaction of ATP←--→ADP.]

Knox, Walter E.

- T. R. Harrison, ed., "Disorders of Amino Acid Metabolism," *Principles of Internal Medicine* (New York: McGraw Hill Book Company, 1962), 746–751.

Krayyer, Otto

- (with E. B. Verney) "Reflecktorishe Beeinflussung des Gehaltes an Acetylcholin in Blute der Coronarvenen," *Naunyn-Shmeideberg's Archiv für experimentelle Pathologie und Pharmakologie*, CLXXX (1935): 75.

Mommaerts, Willfridus F. H. M.

- "Myosin and Adenosinetriphosphate in Muscular Activity," *Science*, CIV (1946): 605.
- (with K. Seraidarian) "A Study of the Adenosine Triphosphate Activity of Myosine and Actinomyosin," *J. Gen. Physiol.*, XXX (1947): 401–422.
- "Reaction between Actinoyosine and Adenosine Triphosphate," *J. Gen. Physiol.*, XXXI (1948): 361–375.

Read, Walter W. C.

- (with D. S. McLaren) "An Unusual Major Fatty Acid Composition in Human Depot Fat," *Nature*, CXCII (1961): 265.
- (with D. S. McLaren) "Fatty Acid Composition of Adipose Tissue: A Study in Three Races in East Africa," *Clinical Science*, XXIII (1962): 247–252.
- (with G. Webber) "The Use of Cobalt 60 for Labeling Snails in the Study of Field Populations," *Annals of Tropical Medicine and Parasitology*, LVI (1962): 206–209.
- (with S. Holmes and G. Drake) "Changes in Body Water and Body Solids in African Adults and their Relation to Nutrition," *Quarterly Journal of Experimental Physiology*, XLVII (1962): 15–31.
- (with S. Kerr) "The Fatty Acid Components of Polyphosphoinositide Prepared from Calf Brain," *Biochimica et Biophysica Acta*, LXX (1963): 477–478.
- (with Z. Audeh) "The Fatty Acid Components of Depot Fat of the Somali Sheep," *Journal of the Science of Food and Agriculture*, XIV (1963): 770–772.
- (with A. Tashjian) "Influence of Diet on Human Milk Fatty Acids," *Proceedings of the Sixth International Congress of Nutrition* (1964): 572.
- (with P. G. Luutz and A. Tashjian) "Human Milk Lipids. I. Changes in Fatty Acid Composition of Early Colostrum. II. The Influence of Dietary Carbohydrate and Fat on the Fatty Acids of Mature Milk. A Study in Four Ethnic Groups. III. Short Term Effects of Dietary Carbohydrate and Fat," *American Journal of Clinical Nutrition*, XVII (1965): 177–187.

Wakid, N. W.

- (with S. E. Kerr) "The Distribution of Posphomonoesterase and Pyrophosphatase in the Particulate Fractions of Dog Cerebrum," *Journal of Histochemistry and Cytochemistry*, III (1955): 75–84.
- "The Measurement of Rotational Speed with Sonometer," *Science*, CXXI (1955): 609–611.
- "Cytoplasmic Fractions of Rat Myometrium. (1) General Description and Some Enzymic Properties," *Biochemical Journal*, LXXVI (1960): 88–95.

- (with D. M. Needham) "Cytoplasmic Fractions of Rat Myometrium. (2) Localization of Some Cellular Constituents in the Pregnant and Ovariectomized States," *Biochemical Journal*, LXXVI (1960): 95–100.
- (with D. M. Needham) "Effect of Estradiol Injection on the Cytoplasmic Fractions of the Myometrium in the Ovariectomized Rat," *Journal of Biophysics, Biochemistry and Cytology*, X (1961): 136–139.
- (with T. E. Mansur and H. M. Sprouse) "Purification and Properties of Sheep Heart Fructokinase," *Federation Proceedings*, XXIV (1965): 2.

Department of Clinical Pathology Laboratory Medicine

A brief history of the blood bank:

Ann Goodenough, MA (biology, University of Rochester School of Medicine and Dentistry), was recruited by the Near East College in New York, NY, in 1946, with a grant of $10,000 to help in establishing a modern blood bank in the Department of Clinical Pathology at AUB. She arrived at AUB in early March, 1947, after having secured equipment in the United States for that purpose. She was greatly helped by Dr. J. J. McDonald (dean), Dr. Whipple, Dr. Bickers, and Dr. Dikran Berberian, as well as Dr. Edmond Shwayri, who was a medical student. The blood bank was operational in 1948.

References:

- The author's personal interview with Ann Goodenough, June 2010.
- Dr. Farid S. Haddad and Dr. Edmond Shwari via e-mail, July 2 2010.
- Dr. Farid S. Haddad's paper on blood transfusion: "Maqalat fy aljirahao," 2003, pp. 73–80.

Abu Haidar, George I.

- (with H. Zellweger and A. J. Dark) "Glycogen Disease of Skeletal Muscle. Report of Two Cases and Review of Literature," *Pediatrics*, XV (1955): 715–732.
- (with F. Chernijoy, A. K. Khachadourian, and S. E. Kerr) "Incorporation of C14 Labelled Glycine and Formate by the Acid-Soluble Guanine and Adenine Nucleotides of Rat Liver," *Journal of Biological Chemistry*, CCXXIV (1957): 707–712.
- (with U. A. S. al-Khalidi, F. Chernijoy, and S. E. Kerr) "A Titimetric Method for the Determination of the Molecular Weight of Small Polynucleotides," *Journal of Biological Chemistry*, CCXXVIII (1957): 487–493.

- (with D. White and J. G. Reinhold) "Spectrophotometric Measurement of Bilirubin Concentrations in the Serum of the Newborn, by the Use of a Microcapillary Method," *Clinical Chemistry*, IV (1958): 211–222.
- (with M. Shahid and N. Abu Haydar) "Thalassemia Hemoglobin E Disease. A Case Report from Quatar (Persian Gulf)," *Man*, CLV (1963): 129.

Alami, Samih Y., chairman

- (with F. C. Kelly) "Influence of Coagulase and Route of Injection on Staphylococcal Bacteria in Mice," *Proceedings of the Society for Experimental Biology and Medicine*, CV (1960): 389–391.

Nassif, Raif E.; chairman (and later) director of the AUB Medical Center

- (Translation from Arabic) "Blood Groups in Determining Paternity. Medico Legal Cases," in Dr. Ghoson Fuad, *Legal Medicine*, 2nd ed. (Beirut: Rihani Publisher, 1965), 817–849.
- "The Incidence of Blood Groups in Lebanon," *Lebanese Medical Journal*, VI (1953): 346–349.
- (with S. A. Attar) "Snake Bite and Snakes in Lebanon," *Lebanese Medical Journal*, VI (1953): 366–375.
- (with W. Long, V. Yonan, and J. G. Reinhold) "Further Studies of Racial Differences in Serum Gamma Globulin Concentrations," *Clinical Chemistry*, II (1956): 238–239.
- (with N. Taleb, and J. Ruffie) Sur la repartition des groups sanguins dans les ethnies Libanaises. C.R. Soc. Biol., Paris, CLV (1961): 1125–1128.

Department of Gynecology and Obstetrics

Abdul Karim, Raja W.

- (with S. D. Larks) "The Normal Fetal Electrocardiogram with a Proposed System of Standardized Terminology," *Institute of Electrical and Electronic Engineering, Transactions on Bio-Medical Electronics*, VIII (1961): 136.
- (with F. Iliya) "Antepartel Diagnosis of Sex," *Lebanese Medical Journal*, XIV (1961): 410–415.
- (with N. S. Assali) "Renal Function in Human Pregnancy. V. Effects of Oxycotin on Renal Hemodynamics and Water and Electrolyte Excretion," *Journal of Laboratory and Clinical Medicine*, CVII (1961): 522–532.
- (with N. S. Assali) "Pressor Response to Angiotonin in Pregnant and Nonpregnant Women," *American Journal of Obstetrics and Gynecology*, CXXXII (1961): 246–251.

- (with G. Iskander) "Acute Hydraminos: Report of Five Cases," *Obstetrics and Gynecology*, XX (1962): 486–489.
- (with L. Abu Nimeh) "Effect of 17-Alpha-Hydroxyprogesterone Caproate on Postpartum Milk Secretion," *Obstetrics and Gynecology*, XX (1962): 636–638.
- (with F. Iliya) "Twin Pregnancy: An Analysis of 162 Cases," *Lebanese Medical Journal*, XV (1962): 80–92.

Ashkar, Philip A.; chairman

- "Functional Sterility," *Journées Médicales de France et de l'Union Française*, II (Mai, 1938).

Bickers, William M., chairman (following Dr. Philip Ashkar's tenure)

- *Outline of Clinical Gynecology* (Springfield, Ohio: Charles C. Thomas Co., 1939; 2nd ed., 1942; 3rd ed., 1947).
- *Premenstrual Tension–A Water Toxicity Syndrome* (monograph) (Springfield, Ohio: Charles C. Thomas Co., 1951).
- *Menorrhalgia–Menstrual Distress* (Springfield, Ohio: Charles C. Thomas Co., 1955).
- *Uterine Contractions in Gynecologic Disorders* (monograph) (Geneva: George & Co., 1955), 52.
- *Gynecologic Therapy* (Springfield, Ohio: Charles C. Thomas Co., 1957).
- *Primary Dysmenorrhea*. A thirty-minute, color, teaching motion picture. Released by the Searle Corporation (1943).
- *Lenorrhea*. A thirty-minute, color, teaching motion picture. Released by the Ciba Corporation (1946).
- (with F. W. Shaw) "Demodex Folliculorum Infestation," *Virginia Medical Monthly*, LXIII (December 1936): 556–557.
- "Pregnancy and Labor in 400 Unmarried Primiparae," *Virginia Medical Monthly*, LXXIII (January 1937): 632–634.
- "Sterility in the Female," *Virginia Medical Monthly*, LXIV (July 1937): 214–216.
- "Case of Pneumococcus Vaginitis Treated with Anti-Serum," *Virginia Medical Monthly*, LXV (February 1938): 104–105.
- "Induction of Ovulation," *Virginia Medical Monthly*, LXVII (1940): 760–762.
- (with R. J. Main) "Patterns of Uterine Motility in Normal Ovulatory and Anovulatory Cycle, after Castration, Coitus and Missed Abortion," *Journal of Clinical Endocrinology and Metabolism*, I (1941): 992–995.
- "Shock from Posterior Pituitary Extract," *Southern Medical Journal*, XXXIV (1941): 1112–1113.
- "Uterine Contractions in Dysmenorrhea," *American Journal of Obstetrics and Gynecology*, XLII (1941): 1023–1030.

- "Intestinal Obstruction Following the Baldy-Webster Suspension of the Uterus," *American Journal of Obstetrics and Gynecology*, XLII (1941): 915.
- "Sulfonamide Suppository in the Treatment of Acute Gonorrhea in Women," *American Journal of Obstetrics and Gynecology*, XLII (1941): 162–163.
- "Near Fatal Reaction to Pregnant Mare Serum," *Journal of Clinical Endocrinology and Metabolism*, I (1941): 852–853.
- "Uterine Contractions in Labor; Effect of Analgesic Drugs," *Virginia Medical Monthly*, LXIX (1942): 15–19.
- "Primary Dysmenorrhea–The Uterine Contraction Patterns," *Virginia Medical Monthly*, LXIX (1942): 423–428.
- "Congenital Syphilis Acquired by Fetus Before Appearance of Chancre in Mother," *Archives of Dermatology and Syphilology*, XLVI (1942): 135–136.
- "Procaine Hydrochloride Infiltration in Obstetrics," *Southern Medical Journal*, XXXV, no. 1 (1942).
- "The Placenta, a Modified Arterio-Venous Fistula," *Southern Medical Journal*, XXXV, no. 1 (1942): 17–20.
- "Effect of Progesterone on Uterine Contractions," *American Journal of Obstetrics and Gynecology*, XLIII (1942): 663–667.
- "A Study of Contractions in Labor Based on Kymographic Records Obtained from an Intrauterine Balloon," *American Journal of Obstetrics and Gynecology*, XLIII (1942): 815–819.
- "Puerperal Uterine Contractions," *American Journal of Obstetrics and Gynecology*, XLIV (1942): 581–584.
- "Leucorrhea, a New Classification and New Approach to Treatment," *Virginia Medical Monthly*, LXX (1943): 135–140.
- "Primary Dysmenorrhea," *Southern Medical Journal*, XXXVI (1943): 192–198.
- "The Ergot Alkaloids," American Journal of Obstetrics and Gynecology, XLVI (1943): 238–244.
- "Post-Operative Retention," *Urologic and Cutaneous Review*, XLVII (1943): 182–185.
- "A Study of the Endometrial Pattern before and after Treatment for Amenorrhea," *American Journal of Obstetrics and Gynecology*, XLVIII (1944): 58–68.
- "Pelvic Abscess Following Artificial Insemination," *American Journal of Obstetrics and Gynecology*, XLVI (1944): 425–426.
- "The Menstrual Irregularities and Their Treatment," *Southern Medical Journal*, XXXVII (1944): 391–399. Reprinted in *Virginia Medical Monthly*, LXXI (1944): 513–521.
- "Clinical Problems Related to Disturbances in Myometrial Physiology," *Dallas Medical Journal*, XXXI (1945): 86–90.
- "Post-Menopausal Nocturia Treated with Testosterone Pellet," *Urologic and Cutaneous Review*, XLIX (1945): 397–398.
- "Non-Effect of Progesterone in Threatened Abortion," *American Journal of Obstetrics and Gynecology*, XLVI (1945).

- "Ethinyl Estradiol in the Treatment of Metrorrhagia," *American Journal of Obstetrics and Gynecology*, LI (1946): 100–103.

- "Dysmenorrhea and Spontaneous Abortion, Physiologic Defeat in Myometrium not Related to Corpus Luteum Failure," *Journal of the Palistine Arab Medical Association*, I (1946): 96–99.

- (with Y. D. Jidejian) "Transplantation of the Ureters into the Rectosigmoid," *Surgery, Gynecology and Obstetrics with International Abstracts of Surgery*, LXXXV (1947): 30–34.

- "The Evolution of Obstetrics and Gynecology in the Near East," *American Journal of Obstetrics and Gynecology*, LIV (1947): 814–819.

- (with P. F. Sahyoun and A. Saadeh) "Granulosa Cell Tumor of the Ovary," *Virginia Medical Monthly*, LXXIV (1947): 509–512.

- "Amenorrhea and Oligomenorrhea, Etiology and Treatment," *American Journal of Obstetrics and Gynecology*, LVI (1948): 893–900.

- (with P. F. Sahyoun and M. Massic) "Vaginal Cervical Smear in the Diagnosis of Uterine Cancer," *Virginia Medical Monthly*, LXXV (1948): 568–574.

- (with M. Woods) "Uterine Muscle Physiology from Laboratory to Bedside, a Treacherous Crossing," *American Journal of Obstetrics and Gynecology*, LVIII (1949): 1099–1108.

- (with R. D. Adams) "Hereditary Stenosis of Aqueduct of Sylvius as Cause of Congenital Hydrocephalus," *Brain*, LXXII (1949): 246–262.

- "Progesterone, a Comparison of Intramuscular, Oral and Sublingual Routes of Administration," *J. Clin. Endor.*, IX (1949): 736–742.

- "Progesterone and Anhydrohydroxyprogesterone—A Comparative Study of Oral Administration," *Journal of Laboratory and Clinical Medicine*, XXXV (1950): 265–270.

- "Postoperative Cervical-Vaginal Healing in Relation to Postoperative Treatment," *American Journal of Obstetrics and Gynecology*, LIX (1950): 1045–1052.

- "Pelvic Autonomic Nervous System–Effect of Electrical Excitation," *Southern Medical Journal*, XLIII (1950): 889–893.

- "The Anti-Pitressin Factor in the Treatment of Dysmenorrhea," *New Engl. J. Med.*, CCXLIII (1950): 645–648.

- "Dysmenorrhea and Pelvic Autonomic System," *Southern Medical Journal*, XLIII (1950): 889–893.

- "Premenstrual Tension: Its Relation to Abnormal Water Storage," *New Engl. J. Med.*, CCXLV (Sept. 1951): 453–456.

- (with M. Woods) "Premenstrual Tension," *Tex. Rep. Biol. Med.*, IX (June 1951): 406–419.

- "Patterns of Uterine Motility in Relation to Spermigration," *Fertil. and Steril.*, II (1951): 342–346.

- "Premenstrual Tension," *New Engl. J. Med.*, (Sept. 20, 1951): 453–456.

- "Premenstrual Tension and Its Relationship to Water Metabolism," *Amer. J. Obstetrics and Gynecology*, LXIV (1952): 587–590.

- "Menstrual Arrhythmias: Oral Estrogen and Progressive Therapy," *Amer. J. Obstetrics and Gynecology*, LXIV (1952): 148–154.
- (with M. Woods) "Premenstrual Distress and What To Do About It," *Amer. J. Nursing*, LII (1952): 1087–1089.
- "Premenstrual Tension–A Neglected Phase of Menstrual Disability," *Sth. Med. J.* (Bgham., Ala.), XLVI (1953): 873–874.
- "Toluidine Blue–An Evaluation in the Treatment of Uterine Bleeding," *American Journal of Obstetrics and Gynecology*, LXVI (1953): 1313–1317.
- "Endometriosis," in *Current Therapy* (Philadelphia: William R. Saunders, 1954), 581–582.
- "The Rh Dilemma," Letter, *Obstetrics and Gynecology*, VII (1956): 713–715.
- "Menstrual Irregularity," *Virginia Medical Monthly*, LXXXIII (1956): 202–205.
- "Uterine Contraction Patterns–Effects of Psychic Stimuli on the Myometrium, *Fertil. and Steril.*, VII (1956): 268–275.
- "Episioperineorrhaphy," *Virginia Medical Monthly*, LXXXIV (1957): 392–395.
- "The Middle East and Our Medical Heritage," *Virginia Medical Monthly*, LXXXV (1958): 531–532.
- "Premenstrual Tension–a Water Toxicity Syndrome," *Virginia Medical Monthly*, LXXXV (1958): 613–615.
- "Uterine Contractions in Gynecologic Disorders," *Scientific Exhibit–Proceedings of Obstetrics and Gynecology Congress*, Geneva (1958).
- "Premenstrual Tension," *Semin. Rep.*, IV (Fall 1959): 10–12.
- "Adam and Eve," guest editorial, *Virginia Medical Monthly*, LXXXVI (1959): 375–376.
- "Endometriosis," *Med. Tms.* (N.Y.), LXXXVII (October 1959): 1317–1319.
- "Sperm Migration and the Emotions," *Proceedings of Pan American Conference on Fertility*, Miami Beach (1960): 159–167.
- "Dysmenorrhea and Menstrual Disability," *Clin. Obstet. Gynec.*, III (1960): 233–240.
- "Sperm Migration and Uterine Contractions," *Fertil. and Steril.*, XI (1960): 286–290.
- "Endometriosis," in *Current Therapy* (Philadelphia: William R. Saunders Co., 1960), 647–649.
- "Therapeutic Abortion," *Lebanese Medical Journal*, XIV (1961): 469–477.
- "François Rabelais, M.D.," *J. Amer. Med. Ass.*, CLXXV (1961): 124–126.
- "Uterine Contractions and the Psyche," *Fertil. and Steril.*, VII (1961): 268–274.
- "Medical Teaching in the Orient," *Virginia Medical Monthly*, LXXXVIII (1961): 387–389.
- "Dismenorrhea–A New Therapy," *Virginia Medical Monthly*, LXXXVIII (1961): 36–39.
- "Leukorrhea," *Lebanese Medical Journal*, XIV (1961): 115–123.
- "American Medicine Abroad," *Current Medical Digest*, XXIX (1962): 51–57.
- "Medicine–East and West," *J. Amer. Med. Ass.*, CLXXXI (1962): 142–150.
- "John Peter Mettauer of Virginia," *J. Amer. Med. Ass.*, CLXXXIV (1963): 870–871.
- "How to Treat Primary Dysmenorrhea," *Consultant* (March 1964).

- "Pelvic Endometriosis," in *Current Therapy* (Philadelphia: William R. Saunders, 1965), 647–649.
- "Pills and Theology," guest editorial, *Virginia Medical Monthly*, XCII (1965): 345–346.
- "Dr. Albert Schweitzer," *J. Amer. Med. Ass.*, CXCIII (1965): 184–185.

Hajj, Samir

- (with B. Brandstater, J. Bitar, M. S. Slim, and H. G. Mishalani) "Congenital Anomalies: Etiology, Diagnosis and Surgical Considerations," *M. E. Medical J.*, II (1965): 24–42.
- (with U. A. S. al-Khalidi and M. H. Shamma'a) "Serum Xanthine Oxidase in Obstetrical Conditions," *American Journal of Obstetrics and Gynecology* (in press).

Khalidy, Mustafa M.; 1920–1947

- Published several ob-gyn papers in Arabic in the local press on motherhood, pregnancy, and delivery, and on diabetes and pregnancy.
- "Progressive Islam," *The Review of Religions*, LV (1961): 244–249.

Mufarrij, Ibrahim H.

- "Trilene Analgesia in Obstetris," *Lebanese Medical Journal*, IX (1956): 670–676.
- "Complications of Abortion," *Lebanese Medical Journal*, X (1957): 123–130.
- (with W. C. Keetel) "Prolapse of Uterus Associated with Pregnancy," *Amer. J. Obstet Gynec.*, LXXIII (1957): 899–903.
- "Pregnancy and Diabetes," *Med. Student Bull.*, I (June 1958).
- "Anencephaly. An Analysis of Anencephalic Births, and a Report of a Case of Repeated Anencephaly," *Obstet. Gynec.*, XXII (1963): 657–661.

Rea, Derek H.

- "Pregnancy Complicated by Cardiac Rheumatic Valvular Disease," *Leb Med. J.*, VI (1953): 351–359.

Suidan, Fayez G.

- (with G. A. Garabedian and R. M. Matossian) "A Correlative Study of Immunological Tests for the Diagnosis of Hydatid Disease," *American Journal of Tropical Medicine and Hygiene*, VIII (1959): 67–71.

Department of Internal Medicine

Abu Faisal, Khalil

- (with A. K. Khachadurian) "Alkaptonuria. Report of a Family with Seven Cases Appearing in Four Generations with Metabolic Studies in One Patient," *J. Chron. Dis.*, VII (1958): 455–465. [**Nassar comment:** This scholarly clinical paper relates the autosomal recessive transmission of alkaptonuria defective gene HGD in four successive family generations. The main clinical feature of the disease is appearance of brown-dark urine on exposure of urine specimen to open air. The abnormality is due to the presence of homogentisic acid, which is an intermediary to tyrosine metabolism resulting in toxic tyrosine. All of this occurs in the liver. Homogentisic acid eventually attacks joints (osteoarthritis), kidneys (stones), and heart (valvular heart disease). There is no known cure. Homogentisin may help temporarily.]
- (with Soni and A. B. Dubois) "The Rate of Intrapulmonary Blood Gas Exchange in Living Animals," *J. Clin. Invest.*, XLII (1963): 16–23.
- (with F. M. Abboud and J. W. Eckstein) "Cardiovascular Responses to Positive Pressure Breathing after Adrenergic Blockage," *Clin. Res.*, XIV (1966): 146–154.

Abu Haidar, Fadlo R.; gastroenterology

- (with G. A. Garabedian and A. Donabedian) "Studies on a Recent Epidemic of Influenza—A Preliminary Report," *Lebanese Medical Journal*, VII (1954): 146–154.
- (J. E. Azar and A. Donabedian) "An Outbreak of Food- Borne Streptococcosis, *Lebanese Medical Journal*, VII (1954): 289–291.
- (G. A. Garabedian and A. Donabedian) "Studies on an Outbreak of Influenza in Beirut, Lebanon," *American Journal of Tropical Medicine and Hygiene*, V (1956): 620–646.

Abu Hydar, Najib

- "Exophthalmos, Digital Clubbing, and Pretibial Mysedema Associated with Hashimoto's Thyroiditis and Hypothyroidism," *Proc. Endocr. Soc. 43rd Meeting* (June 1961).
- "Digital Clubbing and Pretibial Myxedema in Thyroiditis," *Journal of Clinical Endocrinology and Metabolism*, XXIII (1962): 215–217.
- (A. K. Kurban, F. S. Farah, and Ph. Issa) "The Acute Effects of Irradiation on the Alkaline Phosphatase Activity of the Guinea Pig Sebaceous Land," *J. Invest. Derm.*, XXXIX (1962): 3–9.
- (with Munib Shahid) "Sickle Cell Disease in Syria and Lebanon," *Act. Haemat.* (Basel), XXVII (1962): 268–273.

- (with M. Shahid and R. I. Abu Haydar) "Thalassemia Hemoglobin E Disease. A Case Report from Qatar," *Man*, CLV (1963): 109.

Azzam, Samir

- (with A. S. Majaj, J. S. Dining, and S. A. Darby) "Vitamin E Responsive Megaloblastic Anemia in Infants with Protein Calorie Malnutrition," *Amer. J. Nutr.*, XII (1963): 374–375.
- (with J. S. Dining, S. A. Darby, W. J. Shunk, and K. Folkers) "Response of Microcytic Anemia in Children to the Co-Enzyme Q 4-chormanol," *Amer. J. Nutr.*, XIII (1963): 163–172.

Bashour, Fuad A.; cardiology

- (with C. Chidiac) "Pulmonary Hypertension Report of Illustrative Cases with Clinical and Physiological Studies," *Lebanese Medical Journal* (February 1958): 1–10.
- (with D. H. Simmons) "Atrial Septal Defect with Mitral Valvulitis: Clinical and Catheterization Diagnosis," *Ann. Int. Med.* (June 1958): 1194–1204.
- (with P. Winchell) "Some Physiologic Features of Atrial Septal Defect. Observations in 38 Cases," *Amer. J. Cardiol.*, II (1958): 687–693.
- (with I. K. Dagher) "Repeated Extraction of Needles from the Heart," *Lebanese Medical Journal*, XI (1958): 157–166.
- (with J. Khalaf, F. Fuleihan, and I. K. Dagher) "Right Aortic Arch: Report of Two Cases," *Lebanese Medical Journal*, XII (1959) 75–84.

Bellama, Raif A.

- Member of the Faculty of Medicine; his career took him to be a member of the Lebanese government. Published several articles in Arabic medical journals, mainly educational material.
- "War Experiences," *Al Kulliyeh*, VII (January 1920): 33–36.

Chaglassian, Hrant; chairman of the Division of Dermatology

- "Treatment of Leprosy," *Proc. 4th Int. Congr. Trop. Med. Hyg.* (Istanbul) (1953).
- (with J. E. Azar) "Chediac VDRL Blood Test," *Leb. Med. J.* (1954): 138–145.
- (with H. A. Reiman and P. F. Sahyoun) "Primary Amyloidosis. Relationship to Secondary Amyloidosis. Report of a Case," *Arch. Int. Med.* (1954): 673–686. [**Nassar comment:** Authors report on a case of amyloidosis and discuss classification of primary amyloidosis vs. secondary amyloidosis. The main difference, though there is sometimes overlapping between the two diseases, is that primary amyloidosis is not preceded

by a major disease, while in secondary amyloidosis, it is associated with or follows a major disease such as T Bc, or the rheumatoid arthritides or chronic sepsis, with the exception of multiple myeloma amyloidosis, whose pathology involves similar organs as in primary disease, such as the liver, spleen, and kidneys. In a later publication by W. St. Symmers in *J. Clin Path.* (3) (August 9, 1956): 187–211, quoting the work of Reiman, Dr. Symmers reports in 143 cases of primary amyloidosis, the heart was involved with amyloid in 90 percent, G I tract in 70 percent, tongue in 40 percent, kidneys in 35 percent, liver in 35 percent, spleen in 40 percent. These papers are of great importance, because within the last twenty to thirty years, brain amyloid is found in Alzheimer's disease: amyloid plaques are found involving neurons in the brain due to an alpha amyloid protein defect. Is primary amyloidis one cause of Alzheimer's?]

- "A Detailed Report on Venereal Diseases Center of Port-Area," Int. Conf. on the Control of V.D. of Seafarers in Naples (September19–23, 1953).

- "Recent Trends in Venereal Diseases. Gonorrhea, Nonspecific Urethritis, and Chancroid," *The Physician*, V (1956): 36.

- "Recent Trends in V. D. Syphilis," *The Physician*, VIII (1957): 225.

- "Preventive Medicine and Dermatology, Modern Approach," *The Physician*, I (1957): 3.

- [**Nassar comment:** As a notation to the above publications on venereal diseases by Drs. Chaglassian and colleagues, they laid the foundation for modern diagnosis and treatment in Lebanon. Thus, aside from direct dark field visualization of treponema pallidum spirochetes in the exudates from the chankar, the test FTA-ABS yields 100 percent accuracy vs. VDRL (positive only in 70 percent of documented cases), and is confirmed by microhemagglutinin antigen-TP. New approaches to treatment: doxycycline 100 mg bid x14 days or ceftriaxone 2Gm IM or IV daily x14 days. The time-tested approach with benzathine penicillin remains standard: 2.4 million units I.M. weekly for three weeks following a course of aqueous penicillin for CNS syphilis. *Infectious Diseases*, ch. 14, by W. E. Marshall and coworkers in *Mayo Clinic Internal Medicine Concise Textbook*; editor-in-chief, T. M. Habermann and K. Ghosh (Mayo Clinic Scientific Press, 2008), 805–807.]

- "Efficacy of Prednisone in Lichen Planus," *Excerpta Med.* (Amsterdam), sec. XIII, special Congress issue (1957): 129.

- "The Implication of Untoward Reactions to Penicillin," *Lebanese Medical Journal*, XIV (1961): 187–191.

- (with F. S. Farah and A. K. Kurban) "Epidemiology of Skin Diseases in the Middle East," *Proc. XIIth Int. Congr. Derm.*, Washington (1962).

- "The Incidence and Trends of Venereal Diseases in Lebanon 1938–1939; 1945–1960," *Proc. XII Int. Congr. Derm.*, Washington (1962). [Daniel H. Cooper, et al., eds., "Update on Current Treatment of Gonorrhea," *The Washington Manual of Medical Therapeutics*, 32nd edition (USA: Volters Kluver/ Lippincott Williams & Wilkins, 2007), 656.]

- (with A. K. Kurban and F. S. Farah) "Acute Effects of X-Ray Irradiation on the Skin," *Proc XIIth Int. Congr. Derm.*, Washington (1962): 603.

- (with A. K. Kurban and F. S. Farah) "The Treatment of Leishmaniasis," *Minerva Derm.*, XXXIX sup. 1 (1963): 3.
- (with F. S. Farah and A. K. Kurban) "Antibody Valence: Its Role in the Precipitin and Wheal and Erythema Reactions," *Minerva Derm.*, XXXIX sup. 1 (1964): 60.
- (with A. K. Kurban and F. S. Farah) "Alopecia Mucinosa: a Histo-Chemical Study," *Dermatologica* (Basel), CXXIV (1962): 368–405.
- (with A. K. Kurban and F. S. Farah) "Capillary Changes in Some Connective Tissue Diseases," *Dermatologica (Basel)*, CXXIX (1964): 257–265.
- (with F. S. Farah, A. K. Kurban, and S. Y. Alami) "Survey of the Pathogenic Dermatophytes in Lebanon," *Leb Med. J.*, XV (1962): 75–79.
- (with A. K. Kurban and F. S. Farah) "The Evaluation of Palmar Erythema in the Diagnosis of Connective Tissue Diseases," *Lebanese Medical Journal*, XVI (1963): 175–180.
- (with F. S. Farah and A. K. Kurban) "The Effect of Heat on Antibody Activity," *J. of Immunol.*, XCIII (1964): 300–304.
- "Dibenzyl Theylene Diamene Dipenicillen in Early Syphilis," (monograph 1&11), *W.H.O.* (1955).
- "An International Nomenclature of Yaws Lesion," (monograph), *W.H.O.* (1957).
- (with H. K. Homma) *Uber einen Fall von extragenitalern lymphogranuloma inguinale bei einer krankenpflegerin,*" *Wien. Klin. Wschr.* (1935): 464–466.
- (with D. H. Escher) *"Premiers resultants d'une experimentation au Levant du test cutanne' de Frei,*" *Bull. Acad. Med.* (Paris) (1936): 564.
- (with D. H. Escher) "Mycosis—A Preliminary Report about Fungus Infections of the Scalp as Seen at the O.P.D. of AUB," *Journales Medicales de Beyrouth* (1938): 717–720.
- (with D. H. Escher) "Nodular Tuberculous Lymphangitis, Simulating Sporotrichosis," *Journales Medicales de Beyrouth* (1939): 727.
- (with D. H. H. Escher and G. Khabsa) *"Traitment chimio-therapique de la ble'norrhagie par les derives organo-soufre,*" *Journales medicales de Beyrouth* (1939): 750.
- "The Value of Premarital Certificate," *Yeridesarat Heyouhi* (1947).
- "Calciferol Treatment of Leprosy. Preliminary Report of Two Cases," *J. Invest. Derm.* (1948): 303–304.
- (with A. C. Pipkin) "Familial Lentigo," *J. Hered.* (1950): 79– 82.
- (E. Rizk, G. A. Garabedian, A. C. Pipkin) "Studies on Treponema of Bejel—Part I History, Morphologic Characteristics and Staining Properties," *American Journal of Syphilis, Gonorrhea and Venereal Diseases*, XXXV (1951): 201–206.
- (with N. Bustani and H. H. Anderson) "Endemic Treponematosis Balash or Bejel in Saudi Arabia," *Amer. J. Trop. Med. Hyg.*, I (1952): 826–830.

Dowdswell, Roland

- (with J. E. Azar) "Food Poisoning," *Lebanese Medical Journal*, VI (1953): 337–345.
- "An Outbreak of Dysentery in a School," *Lebanese Medical Journal*, VI (1953): 360–365.

Dragatsi, Gregoire

- (with A. K. Kurban, A. I. Shafik, and S. A. Attar) "Echinococcosis of the Heart," *Amer. Heart J.*, XLVI (1953): 764–771.
- (with N. A. Tuqan) "Clinical-Pathological Conference: Epigastric Pain, Melena and Gastric Filling Defect," *Lebanese Medical Journal*, XII (1959): 210–218.

Goodale, Raymond H.

- Several papers in Arabic published in *Al Kuliyah* dealing with fighting cancer, tuberculin testing, and other topics.
- (with H. Krishner) "Biological Tests for Hydatid Disease. A Comparison of the Casoni and Weinberg Tests," *American Journal of Tropical Medicine*, X (1930): 71–76. [**Nassar comment:** This paper shows that clinical research was ongoing. At the time this paper was written, hydatid disease was endemic with sporadic cases reported and surgically treated. The research paper gave the clinicians an insight as to the efficacy of biological testing for the diagnosis of hydatid disease, by comparing the Cassoni skin test and the Weinberg compliment fixation test performed on forty-four cows that had hydatid cysts by examining the cows' organs (post slaughtering of cows at the Abatoire), verifying the presence of hydatid disease. The test value result showed that the Casoni skin test had a higher diagnostic result than the Weinberg.]
- (with H. Krishner) "Geographical Pathology," *New Engl. J. Med.*, CCII (1930): 155.
- "Cystadenoma of the Bladder from Aberrant Prostatic Gland," *Arch. Path.*, VI (1928): 210–214.
- "Hemangio Endothelioma of the Liver," *Arch. Path.*, IX (1930): 528.
- (with H. Krishner) "Racial Tuberculosis in Syria," *Amer. Rev. Tuberc.*, XXI (1930): 223–232.
- (with H. Krishner) "Oxyuris Vermicularis in the Peritoneum," *Arch. Path.*, IX (1930): 631–634.
- (with H. Krishner and L. W. Parr) "The Epidemiology of Diphtheria and Scarlet Fever in the Subtropics with Special Reference to the Syrian States under French Mandate," *J. Prevent. Med.*, IV (1930): 39.
- "Hydatid Disease of the Brain," *American Journal of Tropical Medicine*, XI (1931): 61–64.
- "Racial Tuberculosis in Syria," *Amer. Rev. Tuberc.*, XXXIII (1931): 456–460.

Homma, Hans K.

- (H. A. Yenikomishian) Ein Fall von Spomtano-ruptur desAbsteigen Astes der linken coronarasartene. *Wien. Med. Wschr.* 44 (1933).
- Ueber eine Einfache Methode zur Bestimmung der Bluststromungs Geschwindigkeit in Menschichen Venen. *Wien. Kin. Wschr.*, XLVII (1934): 782.

Hudson, Ellis H.

- "Treponematosis among the Bedouin Arabs of the Syrian Desert," *U.S. Nav. Med. Bull.*, XXVI (1928).

Idriss, H.; see Department of Pediatrics for other published papers by Dr. H. Idriss

- (with L. Giaccai, Department of Radiology) "Osteomyelitis due to Salmonella Infection," *Journal of Pediatrics*, XLI (1952): 73–78.
- (with H. Zellweger) "Encephalopathy in Salmonella Infections," *Amer. J. Dis. Child.*, LXLIX (1960): 770–777.

Kegel, Richard F. C.

- "The Diagnosis of Pulmonary Tuberculosis," *Rev. Med. Lib.*, I (1948): 159–161.

Khayat, George B.; professor emeritu; preceded Dr. Riad Tabbarah as chairman of the Department of Medicine

[**Nassar comment:** Coauthor with Dr. Kenneth Turner of a clinical research paper on the relationship of cholesterol and hypothyroidism in rabbits. This experimental research work was published in 1933 way ahead of its time before the interest in atherosclerosis, hypercholesterolemia, and its treatment became a hot topic in medicine. The title of the paper is "Studies on the Prevention of Cholesterol; Atherosclerosis in Rabbits. II. The Influence of Thyroidectomy upon the Protective Action of Potassium Iodide," *J. Exp. Med.*, LVIII (1933): 127–135. This paper is a continuation of what the authors reported in a paper I., that whole thyroid replacement and potassium iodide are effective in preventing atherosclerosis in rabbits fed cholesterol. Conclusion of their study: "Thyroidectomy in itself does not cause a rise in blood cholesterol or the development of atherosclerosis in young rabbits." With or without thyroid gland, feeding high cholesterol diets results in hypercholesterolemia and atherosclerosis. Finally, potassium iodide prevents hypercholesterolemia and atherosclerosis of rabbit aorta, but not so in the absence of thyroid glands.]

Krishner, Harold

- (with L. W. Parr) "Hemolytic Transfusion Fatality with Donor and Recipient in the Same Blood Group," *J. Amer. Med. Ass.*, CXCVIII (1932): 47.
- Infectious diseases papers, Internal Medicine, Faculty of Medicine of the American University of Beirut.

Makari, Jack

- "Intradernal Test in Malaria. I," *Transactions of the Royal Society of Tropical Medicine and Hygiene*, XLIK (1946): 23–29.
- "The Cephalin-Flocculation Test in Chronic Malaria and Its Relation to Endemicity," *J. Trop. Med.*, XLIX (1946): 92–94.
- "Cephalin-Flocculation Test in the Selection of Pre-Icteric Infective Hepatitis and the Prevention of Homologus Serum Jaundice," trans., Roy. Soc., *Trop. Med. Hug.*, XXXIX (1946): 540.
- "Intradermal Test in Malaria. II and III," *J. Trop. Med.*, XLIX (1946): 47–57.
- "The Cephalin-Flocculation Test in Malaria," *British Medical Journal*, I (1946): 272–275.
- "Congenital Malaria," *Brit. Med. J.*, I (1946): 662.

Nucho, Nimeh K.; 1903–1949, professor emeritus

- Wrote several papers in Arabic published in the *Al Kulliya Journal* dealing with prevention of TB, treatment of diabetes withinsulin, newer concept in the prevention of TB in the Near East, including a paper on pleurodesis for lung TB infection.

Oliver, Kenneth S.

- (with E. L. Turner) "Acute Edema of the Larynx Complicating Measles," *J. Amer. Med. Association*, CI (1933): 1807.

Parr, Leland

- "Intestinal Spirochetes," *Journal of Infectious Diseases*, XXXIII (1923): 369–383.
- (with B. F. Avery) "The Relationship of the Dick Test to the Prevalence of Scarlet Fever in Grand Lebanon."
- "Modified Wright's Technic for the Standardization of Vaccines," *J. Lab. Clin. Med.*, XIII (1928): 767–768.
- "Negative Results Obtained in the Attempt to Relate Tuberculosis Susceptibility on Resistance to a Particular Blood Group," *J. Prevent. Med.*, III (1929): 237–243.
- "Studies in Isohemagglutination," *Journal of Immunology*, XVI (1929): 99–107.
- "Is Immunity to Scarlet Fever a Factor in Puerperal Sepsis?" *J. Prevent. Med.*, IV (1930): 105–108.
- "On Isohemagglutination, the Hemolytic Index, and Heterohemagglutination," *Journal of Infectious Diseases*, XLVI (1930): 173–185.
- (with R. H. Goodale and R. H. Krishner) "The Epidemiology of Diphtheria and Scarlet Fever in the Subtropics with Special Reference to the Syrian States under French Mandate," *J. Prevent. Med.*, IV (1930): 39–48.

Pipkin, Alan C.

- (with G. A. Garabedian and J. E. Azar) "An Intensive Treatment Regimen of Visceral Schistosomiasis with Fuadin," *American Journal of Tropical Medicine*, XXIX (1949): 595–604.
- (with H. T. Chaglassian) "Familial Lentigo," *J. Hered.*, XLI (1950): 79–82.
- (with E. Rizk, G. A. Garabedian, and H. T. Chaglassian) "Studies on Treponemes of Bejel. Part I. History, Morphologic, Characteristics and Staining Properties," *Am. J. Syph.*, XXXV (1951) 201–206.

Plimpton, Calvin; chairman of Department of Medicine, Faculty of Medicine American University of Beirut

- "Problems in Hypercalcemia," *Proc. VIIth M.E.M.A.* (1957): 241.
- "Management of Addison's Disease with Reference to Use of 9 Alpha-Fluorohydrocortisone," *Proc., M.E.M.A.* (1957): 265.
- "Management of Uncomplicated Diabetes Mellitus," *NY St. J. Med.* (1957).
- (with F. Fuleihan) "Chlorpropamide and Diabetes," *Ann. NY Acad. Sci.*, LXXIV (1959).

Reiman, Hobart A., chairman of Department of Medicine

- "Viral and Bacillary Dysentery. A Dual Epidemic," *J. Med. Assoc.*, CXLIX (1952): 1619–1623.
- (with J. Moadie') "Periodic Abdominalgia (Armenian Disease)," *Leb. Med. J.*, VI (1953): 24–28.
- "Infectious Diseases," *Arch. Intern. Med.*, XCI (1953): 353–388.
- "The Abuse of Antibiotics in Medical Practice," *Lebanese Medical Journal*, VI (1953): 88–92.
- "A Periodic Disease," *Arch. Intern. Med.*, XCII (1953): 494–506.
- (with J. Moadie, S. Semerdjian, and P. H. Sahyoun) "Periodic Disease and Pathology. Report of 72 Cases," *J. Amer. Med Association*, CLIV (1954): 1254–1259. [**Nassar comment:** This clinical research paper with pathologic evidence is a valuable informative paper on the incidence of periodic disease of unknown etiology in seventy-nine cases studied in Lebanon over a period of five years. The affected cases were predominantly Armenians (only seventy-two patients were documented ethnically: forty-nine patients were of Armenian background and twenty-three patients were Arabs). Numerous instances of periodic disease were noted in relatives attesting to its genetic connection. The age onset ranged from before twelve years to fifty-six years. Symptoms and signs of the disorder varied from periodicity of abdominal pains distention, peritonitis, arthralgias, temperature ranged from 38 degrees C to 40 degrees C. with leucocytosis (11,000–26,000), oliguria, or polyurea. Pathologically when appendectomy (eleven

cases) or cholycystectomy (six cases) were done, the serosal surfaces were inflamed with leucocyte infiltrates. There is a suggestion from Dr. Rieman and coworkers that periodic disease may have a relationship to connective tissue disease.]

- (with P. F. Sahyoun, and H. T. Chaglassian) "Primary Amyloidosis, Relationship to Secondary Amylodosis. Report of a Case," *Arch. Intern. Med.*, XCIII (1954): 673–686.
- [Nassar comment: could primar amyloidosis be one cause of Alzheimer's Disease?]
- "Adrenocortical Steroids in the Treatment of Infectious Diseases," *Proc VIIIth M.E.M.A.* (1958): 95–105.

Rubeiz, G. A.; cardiology

- (with F. S. Farah) "Pheochromocytoma: Diagnosis and treatment Illustrated by a Case Report," *Lebanese Medical Journal*, X (1957): 335–345.
- "Paroxysmal Atrial Tachycardia with Block, a Manifestation of Digitalis Toxicity," *Lebanese Medical Journal*, XII (1960): 334–343. [**Nassar comment:** Of the five patients with PAT with block reported by the author, one patient was under my care. All the patients were treated with KCL while withholding digoxin and diuretics in the presence of normal renal function. All five patients reverted to normal regular sinus rhythm. Pronestyl is used with impaired renal function.]
- "The Role of the Cardiologist in Open Heart Surgery," *Arab. Med. J.*, 1 (1961): 14–15.
- (with A. A. Salem) "Analysis of the Cardiac Rhythm during Pre- and Postoperative Periods in Patients Who Underwent Mitral Commissurotomy," *Leb. Med. J.*, 14(1) (1961): 404–409. [**Nassar comment:** Eighty-eight patients were studied. It appeared that those patients with preoperative premature atrial or nodal beats were more prone to develop atrial fibrillation postoperatively. The overall incidence of atrial fibrillation in the eighty-eight patients analyzed was 32 percent. Of those, 14 percent reverted to regular sinus rhythm within two weeks postoperatively. Preoperative digoxin did not prevent the occurrence of atrial fibrillation in the postoperative period. At the time of the conclusion of the study, I was part of the team. At that period in history, quinidine was the drug of choice or pronestyl, if the former did not work. However, newer drugs are now being tried. At AUB, thanks to Drs. G. Fawaz, G. A. Rubeiz, and Riad Tabbara, there were many clinical notations of success with the use of quinidine for atrial fibrillation in rheumatic heart disease, in selected cases, in the 1950s through 1970. On many occasions, digoxin was used alone for rate control. Warfarin was also part of the treatment.]
- (with M. E. Nassar) "The Significance of the Post Extra Systolic T Wave Changes," *Lebanese Medical Journal*, XIV (1961): 181–186. [**Nassar comment:** The clinical significance of this change in the T wave following a normal PQRST wave was found to have a close correlation with presence of heart disease, coronary artery disease being the most frequent heart disease, suggesting that such T wave phenomenon may be a predictor of coronary artery disease, possibly even in asymptomatic patients. This

paper may alert physicians to the clinical significance of post extra T wave change and its relation to underlying, unrecognized coronary heart disease.]

- (with S. Kaid Bey) "Atrial Flutter with 1:1 A-V Conduction," *Amer. J. Cardiol.*, VII (1961): 733–736.

- (with M. H. Shamma'a) "Acute Pancreatitis and Electrocardiographic Evidence of Acute Myocardial Infarction," *American Journal of Medicine*, XXXII (1962): 827–830. [**Nassar comment:** The authors have reported on a patient with acute "embolic?" pancreatitis with associated electrocardiographic (EKG) changes of myocardial infarction. They review the scant literature on this subject, stating that several upper gastrointestinal conditions, from gall bladder disease to acute pancreatitis to peptic ulcer disease to esophageal disease, demonstrate arrhythmias or changes compatible with infarction, though the exact mechanism of this association is not clear. The reported patient had a history of atrial fibrillation and periods of regular sinus rhythm. On emergency admission with the diagnosis of acute pancreatitis, he was in atrial fibrillation with associated changes of myocardial infarction in the EKG. Animal experiments on dogs with injection of taurocholate and/or bile into the pancreatic duct showed EKG changes compatible with infarct, but at autopsy the coronary arteries were found to be normal (J. Gottesman, et al., "Changes in the Electrocardiogram Induced by Pancreatitis," *J.A.M.A.* 123:892 (1943); Pollock, et al., "Electrocardiographic Changes in Acute Pancreatitis," *Surg* 40 (1956): 951. If I may, with authors' permission, since I was the resident who attended to the patient and admitted him to the hospital, I would like to suggest a mechanism to explain some of these associations of acute pancreatitis and the EKG. It is possible that it was caused by a small embolus from the left atrium because of atrial fibrillation lodged in the pancreatic artery or tributary, causing the pancreatitis. Also the same could have occurred to a branch of the coronary arteries. However, in the absence of the latter, the associated EKG changes may be explained on spasm of the coronary artery, clinically known as Prinzmetal angina. The latter may show normal coronary artery and the spasm is reversible.]

- (with N. G. Saab) "Hemodynamic Study in a Case of Progressive Muscular Dystrophy," *Amer. J. Cardiol.*, X (1962): 890–893.

- "Experiences with Left Heart Catheterization," *IXth M.E.M.A. Proc.* (1959): 58–73.

- "Functional Tricuspid Regurgitation in Mitral Valve Disease," *Proceedings of the 10th Middle East Medical Assembly* (1960): 440–450. [**Nassar comment:** The conclusion of this paper is that pure mitral valve stenosis, untreated, causes pulmonary hypertension with resultant right ventricular dilatation, with dilatation of the ring of tricuspid valve causing the functional systolic murmur heard at the lower left sternal border that increases with respiration, distinct from the opening snap (o s) and diastolic rumble of mitral stenosis at the cardiac apex. There is, in my opinion, a nebulous, grade 1, systolic murmur at the cardiac apex due to the stiffened "fish mouth" mitral valve opening in pure mitral valve stenosis, noted at postmortem specimens or confirmed by the bloodstream jet on the index finger felt during ventricular systole by the cardiac surgeon before finger mitral commissurotomy procedure. References: (a) verbal comments by the cardiac surgeon; and (b) the description of pure mitral valve stenosis as "fish mouth" described in W. A. D. Anderson, eds., *Pathology*, 2nd ed. (St. Louis: C. V. Mosby Co., 1953), 461. This faint systolic murmur has not been noted in the medical literature. A more complete discussion is in chapter 4. So, in essence there are four sounds in pure mitral stenosis: the opening snap; followed by the classical diastolic rumble; the functional systolic murmur of tricuspid insufficiency; and the soft, difficult-to-hear (by the stethoscope) grade 1 systolic murmur at the cardiac apex, with regular sinus rhythm during cardiac auscultation.]

- (with M. S. Slim, H. D. Yacoubian, J. L. Wilson, and L. Ghandour- Mnaymneh) "Successful Bilateral Reimplantation of the Canine Lungs," *Surgery*, LV (1964): 676– 683. [**Nassar comment:** This important clinical research paper leads one to speculate about the future possible relationship to the research on lung transplantation for chronic obstructive lung disease and lung fibrosis.]

- (with M. E. Nassar and I. K. Dagher) "Study of the Right Atrial Pressure Pulse in Functional Tricuspid Regurgitation and Normal Sinus Rhythm," *Circulation*, XXX (1964): 190–193. [**Nassar comment:** The conclusion of this hemodynamic study of the right atrial pulse was that the A-c-X descent V and Y descent are recorded ordinarily to evaluate the degree of "organic" tricuspid regurgitant disease murmur. However, this study demonstrated that the right atrial pulse pressure curve is preserved in functional tricuspid regurgitation. Hence the jugular venous pressure pulse recording may be used clinically to differentiate functional from organic tricuspid valve disease. This work was cited as reference by Braunwald's *Heart Disease Textbook* (1990) and in *Clinical Phonocardiography and External Pulse Recording* by Morton E. Tavel (Year Book Publishers Inc.: Chicago, 1972): 50, 305.]

- (with M. E. Nassar and A. Touma) "Correlation of the Two-Step Exercise Test and the Hemodynamic Findings in Patients with Mitral Stenosis," *Amer. Heart J.*, LXVII (1964): 311–315. [**Nassar comment:** Both pulmonary hypertension secondary to moderately severe mitral valve stenosis may be assumed to compromise coronary artery blood flow with EKG changes of coronary artery disease. However, according to Drs. P. D. White and P. Wood, in active untreated rheumatic heart disease, arteritis of the coronary arteries may occur and thus in the presence of severe mitral stenosis may be an added factor in compromising coronary artery blood flow, causing angina pectoris. Briefly, though serendipity is hard to come by in science, this study affords such a finding not sought after. Currently, there is a debate in cardiovascular medicine as to the etiology of the coronary artery syndrome: is the symptomatic atheromatous plaque caused by an inflammatory process, or the result of it? C-reactive protein (CRP) was found to be positive (normal value =< 0.8 mg/dl). (Reference: L. G. Gomella, MD, FACS; and S. A. Haist, MD, MS, FACP, "Clinician's Pocket Reference," *McGraw Hill Medical* (2007), 53–54, 210.) Now, CRP is a nonspecific test found positive in infectious diseases and in the rheumatological diseases, such as acute or active rheumatic fever or rheumatic heart disease, valvulitis, arteritis, secondary to a recent beta-hemolytic streptococcus infection, group A Lancefield classification.

It is of great interest to note that in the 1950–1960s period, Drs. John L. Wilson, G. A. Rubeiz, and I were involved in an NIH grant study of rheumatic heart disease patients in Lebanon. CRP was routinely measured along with sedimentation rate and antistreptolysin-O titer (ASL-O) to verify specifically the etiology that Beta hemolyticus strep caused the elevated CRP and sedimentation rate. There was a strong correlation of about 90 percent between the active rheumatic disease process and the laboratory tests of CRP and ASL-O and ESR. Rising ASL-O titer confirmed b-hemolytic strep infection. Hence, the etiology of the inflammatory process of the atheromatous plaque in coronary artery syndrome may be associated as it relates to group A streptococci infections in patients with clinical or subclinical rheumatological disease.]

- "Recent Advances in Primary Myocardial Disease," *Lebanese Medical Journal*, XVII (1964): 37–41.
- (with M. Hajj and A. Touma) "Successful Use of External Electrical Cardioversion in the Treatment of Ventricular Fibrillation Caused by Quinidine," *Amer. J. Cardiology*, XVI (1965): 118–121. [**Nassar comment:** I happened to be on Medicine 1 Pavilion on a Saturday afternoon, off duty and preparing to leave, when the nurse called me on a patient who had lost consciousness while being treated for atrial fibrillation with quinidine. I instituted CPR and the patient revived momentarily and the EKG showed again atrial fibrillation and runs of ventricular wide complex beats, and then patient went into ventricular fibrillation. I defibrillated him with the assistance of Dr. A. Touma (cardiology fellow) and the patient revived, fully conscious with normal neurological findings. The patient also had received epinephrine and normal saline IV, which are recommended for treatment of quinidine toxicity. This paper was written up without acknowledging my role in reviving patient with quinidine toxicity cardiac arrest.]
- (with Mahir R. Awdeh, Fuad Y. Jubran, and Ibrhim K. Dagher) "Successful Surgical Repair of Ruptured Posteromedial Papillary Muscle," *Lebanese Medical Journal* 27 (1) (1974): 17–36.
- (with S. Isa and F. Jubran) "Intracardiac Catheterization. A One-Year Experience at the American University Medical Center," *Lebanese Medical Journal* 25 (4) (1972): 269–284.
- "Takayasu's Disease," *Lebanese Medical Journal* 26 (2) (1973): 119– 126.

Salem, Antoun

- (with A. Tashijian, and M. H. Shamma'a) "Oral Antibiotics and Serum Cholesterol Level in Man," *Clin. Med.* LXX, 1963, 776–779.

Schinazi, Lewis A. (infectious Disease and parasitology)

- (with C.W. Schwabe) Distribution of protonoephridial flame cells in larval Echinococcous Granulosus. J. parasit., XLIV, 1958, 558.
- (with C.W. Schwabe and A. Kilejian) Host-parasite relationships in Echinococcosis. II- Age resistance to secondary Echinococcosis in the white mouse. J.Trop. Med. Hyg. VIII, 1959, 29–36.
- (with C.W. Schwabe and A. Kilejian) Host Parasite relationships in Echinococcosis. V. Histochemical observations on Echinococcus granulosus. J Parast. LXVII, 1961, 181–185.

Scott, Virgil C., chairman of Department of Medicine, Faculty of Medicine, AUB

- "Q Fever in Lebanon; Report of Two Cases," *Lebanese Medical Journal*, X (1957): 188–200.
- Cecil & Loeb, eds.,"Lymphogranuloma Venereum," *Textbook of Medicine*, 9th ed. (W. B. Sauders and Company, 1955), 52–55.

Senekjian, Harutune A.

- (with E. W. Dennis) "On the relationship of Opsonization to Somatic and Flagellar Agglutination by the Blood of Vaccinated Individuals," *Am. J. Hyg.*, XXVI (1937): 11–26.
- (with E. W. Dennis) "Typhoid Leukocidin," *Proceedings of the Society for Experimental Biology and Medicine*, XXXVI (1937): 61–63.
- (with E. W. Dennis) "Recent Experimental Observations on the Pathogenesis of Typhoid Fever," *J. Egypt. Med. Assoc.*, XXI (1938): 738.
- (with E. W. Dennis) "On the Leukocidal Activity of Typhoid Filtrate," *Am. J. Hyg.* XXX (1929): 21–36.
- (with E. W. Dennis) "A Leukocidal Toxin Extracted from Typhoid Bacilli," *Am. J. Hyg.*, XXX (1939): 103–111.

Shahid, Munib J.; chairman of Hematology and Oncology, Faculty of Medicine, AUB

[**Nassar comment:** In 1961-1962, *The American Journal of Medicine* published clinical research on bone marrow transplant for the treatment of leukemia. Dr. Farid Hourani, an AUB graduate physician, was working in a clinical hematology lab in Philadelphia, USA, and was featured as one of the proponents of research on bone marrow and was a coauthor in one of the papers in *The American Journal of Medicine*. Dr. Shahid and I, in the residency program, discussed the papers in a medical conference. Later on, Dr. Hourani was invited to participate in lecturing at the AUB Faculty of Medicine.]

- (with H. A. Yenikomshian) "Typhoid Fever in Inoculated and Noninoculated Persons," *Journe'es Medicales Libanais de Beyrouth* (May 1938) 241–247.
- "The Use of Nitrogen Mustard in the Neoplastic Diseases of the Bone Marrow," *Rev. Med. Liban.* I. (1961?): 45–51.
- (with E. Stephan) "Perarterite noueuse-Maladie de Kussmaul." *Rev. Med. Moy. Or.*, VI (1949): 295–303.
- ACTH et cortisone en hematologie. Rev. Med. Moy. Or., XI (1954): 279–291.
- Quelques considerations sur le favisme au Liban. Rev. Med. Moy. Or., (1960): 83–86.
- (with N. A. Abu-Haydar) "Sickle-Cell Diseases in Syria and Lebanon," *Acta Haemat., Basel*, XXVII (1962): 268–273.
- (with G. I. Abu-Haydar, and N. A. Abu-Haydar) "Thalassemia Hemoglobin E Disease. A Case Report from Quatar," *Persian Gulf, Man.*, CLV (1963): 129.
- "Hemoglobinopathies in Lebanon and Arab Countries," *Proc. IXth Congr. European Soc. Haemat.*, II (1963): 496–500.
- "Iron Absorption in Thalassemia," *Abstr. IXth Congr. Int. Soc. Haemat.* (Stockholm, 1964).

SHAMMA'A, Munir H.; gastroenterology

[**Nassar comment:** Dr. Shamma'a is recognized for his clinical studies on hepatitis A and B, and what was later found to be hepatitis C. Also Dr. Shamma'a is recognized in his clinical work and published work on certain important liver function tests in the diagnosis of liver disease. Also, the paper on nitric oxide and the clinical problem of the hepato renal syndrome is of special importance. The published papers on xanthine oxidase in acute liver injury and in cirrhosis deserve special mention. Moreover, the paper on the diagnosis of enteric fever, malabsorptive conditions of the small intestine, and liver cirrhosis with use of the D-Xylose test is a classic.]

- "Medical Problems in Lebanon," *New Engl. J. Med.*, CCLVII (1957): 218–221.
- (with E. B. Benedict) "Esophageal Web. Report on 58 Cases with an Attempt at Classification," *New Engl. J. Med.*, CCLIX (1957): 378–384.
- (with R. A. Joske and G. D. Drummey) "Intestinal Malabsorption Following Temporary Occlusion of Superior Mesenteric Artery," *Amer. J. Med.*, XXV (1958): 449–455.
- "The Present Status of Hepatic Coma," *Lebanese Medical Journal*, XII (1959): 464.
- (with S. A. Ghazanfar) "D-Xylose Test in Enteric Fever, Cirrhosis and Malabsorptive States," *British Medical Journal*, II (1960): 836–838.
- (with G. A. Rubeiz) "Acute Pancreatitis with Electrocardiographic Evidence of Myocardial Infarction," *Amer. J. Med.*, XXXII (1962): 827–830.
- (with J. Sommerville) "Bile Acid and Cholesterol Metabolism," *Lebanese Medical Journal*, XVI (1963): 75–86.

- (with A. Salem and A. Tashjian) "Oral Antibiotics and Serum Cholesterol Level in Man," *Clin. Med.*, LXX (1963) 776–779. [**Nassar comment:** The result of the study giving sulphalidine and tetracycline phosphate to nine students on a controlled diet with serum cholesterol determination over a period of nine days revealed no change in their cholesterol. Similarly the clinical experiment protocol was repeated for seven students on a regular diet receiving the same antibiotics, and revealed no change or alterations in their serum cholesterol.]
- (with U. S. al-Khalidi) "Dietary Carbohydrates and Serum Cholesterol in Man," *American Journal of Clinical Nutrition*, XIII (1963): 194–196.
- (with U. S. al-Khalidi) "Uptake of Cholesterol by Segments of Small Intestine of Rat," *American Journal of Physiology*, CCVII (1964): 33–36.
- (with M. Uwaydah) "The Treatment of Typhoid Fever with Ampicillin," *Lancet*, I (1964): 1242–1243. [**Nassar comment:** Ampicillin treatment of typhoid fever was compared to chloramphenicol treatment in controlling the disease clinically. It was found that the ampicillin treated typhoid patients was as effective as the chloramphenicol group. The former treatment took nine days to control the infection while the latter took seven days.]
- (with U. S. al-Khalidi, S. Nasrallah, and A. K. Khachadurian) "A Sensitive Method for the Determination of Xanthine Oxidase Activity," *Clinical Chemistry Acta*, XI (1965): 72–77.
- (with L. Ghandur- Mnaymneh) "Clinical-Pathology Conference," *Lebanese Medical Journal*, XVII (1964): 141–152.
- (with U. S. Khalidi) "Serum Xanthine Oxidase Determination and Hepatic Disease," *Lebanese Medical Journal*, XVII (1954): 231–232. [**Nassar comment:** This paper is discussed with U. S. Khalidi previously.]
- (with V. Kilejian, and Z. Ajans) "Bromsulphthalein–BSP, Physiology, Biochemistry and Clinical Applications," *Lebanese Medical Journal*, XVII (1964): 217–226.
- (with S. Nasrallah, A. K. Khachadurian, U. A. S. al-Khalidi, and T. Chaglassian) "Serum Xanthine Oxidase. A Sensitive Test of Acute Liver Injury," *Gastroenterology*, XLVIII (1965): 226–230.
- (S. Nasrallah, and U. A. S, al-Khalidi) "Serum Xanthine Oxidase in the Differential Diagnosis of Jaundice," *J. Lab. Med.* (in press).
- (with U. A. S. al-Khalidi and R. Jeha) "The Comparative Sensitivity of Serum Xanthine Oxidase, Glutamic Oxalometic, and Glutamic Pyruvic Transaminases in Carbon Tetrachloride Induced Hepatic Necrosis in Sheep," *Biochimica et Biophysica Acta* (in press).
- (with S. Hajj and U. A. S. al-Khalidi) "Serum Xanthine Oxidase in Obstetrical Conditions," *American Journal of Obstetrics and Gynecology* (in press).
- (with S. S. D-Jalbut, K. Khuri, and I. Salti) "VIPOMA of the Small Intestine," *Arab J. Med.*, vol. 1, no. 6 (1974): 5–8.

- (with A. Mouradian) "Liver Cirrhosis in Middle Eastern Population. A Comparative Study of Clinical and Histological Features," *Arab J. Med.*, vol 1, no. 2 (1973): 7–11.
- (with S. M. Nasrallah and V. Nassar) "Genetic and Immunological Aspects of Familial Chronic Active Hepatitis (Type B)," *Gastroenterology*, vol. 75, no. 2 (1978): 302–306.

Shuman, John

- "A hospital in Syria," *Am. J. Nursing*, XXIV (1924): 492.
- "Syria and the American University," *Med. Herald* (July 1924): 158.
- "The Resistance of Malaria to Quinine," *J. Amer. Med. Association*, LXXXII (1924): 1382.
- (with W. D. Cruikshank) "Amoebic Colitis with Perforation," *Med. Herald* (December 1922).
- "Acute Epidemic Encephalitis," *Calif. West. Med.* (July 1924).
- "Dengue," *J. Amer. Med. Association*, LXXXII (1924): 737–738.
- "Hydatid Brain Cyst," *Med. J. Rec.* (July 1924).
- (with W. D. Cruikshank) "Duodenal Intestinal Obstruction Secondary to Gastric Polyp and Intussusceptions due to Multiple Teniae Saginata," *N. Y. Med. J.* (June 1923).
- "Medical Work in Syria," *Med. J. Rec.* (April 1, 1925).
- "The Aim of the Medical Student," *Al kulliyah*, IX (December 1922). Reprinted in *Med. Times*, N.Y., LIII (December 1925).

Shwayri, Edmond; nephrology, Department of Medicine Faculty of Medicine, AUB

- (with E. Rizk, and G. A. Garabedian) "Studies on the Treponemes of Bejel—Part II Transmission to Rabbits and Observation on the Course of Experimental Infection," *Am. J. Syph.*, XXXV (1951): 207–215.
- (with R. Cotran, K. Abu Feisal, and F. S. Farah) "Viral Hepatitis. I. Review and Report of 104 Cases of Acute Icteric Hepatitis," *Lebanese Medical Journal*, VIII (1955): 37–55.
- (with N. Tutunji) "Periodic Disease. Report of a Case of Recurrent Abdominal and Thoracic Pain with Synchronous Gross Hematuria," *Arch. Intern. Med.* (1955): 337–340.
- (with N. S. Bricker, J. B. Reardan, D. Kellog, J. P. Merrill, and J. H. Holmes) "An Abnormality in Renal Function Resulting from Tract Obstruction," *Am. J. Med.* (1957): 554–564. [**Nassar comment:** Four patients were studied who had renal failure secondary to mechanical urinary tract obstruction with clinical measurements of renal urinary function post relieve of urinary obstruction. Results are briefly summarized here: GFR, sodium chloride excretion, and urinary volume were measured for several days up to several months. The main findings were marked daily polyurea of 4.5l to 15l. The main defect causing large volume osmotic diuresis of sodium chloride was attributed to lack of controlled reabsorption of sodium chloride in the proximal tubules, which suggested some kind of suppression for reabsorption. This type of

obstructive uropathy with relief had several effects on renal function similar clinically to advanced Bright's disease.]

- "Certain Aspects of the Management of Renal Failure," *Lebanese Medical Journal*, X (1957): 317–326. Reprinted in *Proc. VIIth M.E. M. A.* (1957): 136–145.
- (with D. Ingvar, F. S. Haddad, S. Cronquist, F. Sabra, and N. Tuqan) "Clinical Pathological Conference—Brain Abscess and Uremia," *Middle East Medical Journal*, I (1962): 79–90.
- (with R. Damidian, and N. S. Bricker) "On the Existence of Non–Urine Forming Nephrons in the Diseased Kidney of the Dog," *J. Lab. Med.*, LXV (1965): 26–39.

Tabbara, Riad A.; cardiology chair

[**Nassar comment**: Dr. Tabbara has also published a paper on Chagas' Disease (of the heart). It is unavailable at present.]

- (with D. Kazzaz) "The Effect of Reprodal (Fuadin) on the Electrocardiogram of the Dog," *Amer. J. Trop. Med.*, XXXI (1951): 510–513. [**Nassar comment:** The study of the effect of Reprodal on the electrocardiogram of a dog's heart was undertaken to show that Reprodal had no untoward effect on the electrocardiogram to reinforce its safety in its therapeutic application for the treatment of vesical schistomiasis. Refer to the next article on this topic.]
- (with J. E. Azar) "A Report of the Intensive Treatment of Vesical Schistosomiasis," *Transactions of the Royal Society of Tropical Medicine and Hygiene*, XLV (1951): 383–388.
- (with J. L. Wilson) "The Surgical Treatment of Heart Disease," *Lebanese Medical Journal*, IX (1958): 131–180.
- (with N. A. Tuqan) "Clinical–Pathological Conference: Transposition of the Great Vessels, Inter-Auricular and Inter-Ventricular Septal Defects," *Lebanese Medical Journal*, XI (1958): 317–332.
- Refer to his coauthorship with Dr. John L. Wilson; published a treatise on surgical treatment of heart disease.

Turner, Edward; chairman of the Department of Medicine, AUB (already cited above)

Watson, John M.

- "Clinical Investigation on the Treatment of Urinary Bilharziasis, Part III. Vitamin A.," *J. Trop. Med.*, LV (1952): 128–135.
- (with R. Mackeith) "The Comparative Efficiency of Various Techniques for the Diagnosis of Threadworm Infection," *Arch. Dis. Childh.*, XXVII (1952): 526–532.
- "Bilharzia in South Persia," *Transactions of the Royal Society of Tropical Medicine and Hygiene*, XLVII (1953): 49–55.

Yenikomshian, Hovsep A.; professor emeritus, chairman of the Department of Medicine, AUB

- (with D. A. Berberian) "The Occurrence and Distribution of Human Helminthiasis in Syria and the Lebanon," *Arch. Dis. Childh.*, XXVII (1934): 425–435.
- "Non-Alcoholic Cirrhosis of the Liver in Lebanon and Syria," *J. Mer. Ass.*, CIII (1934): 660–661.
- "A Case of Septicaemic Plague Simulating Pernicious Malaria," *Indian Med. Gaz.*, LXX (1935): 508–509.
- (with H. K. Blake) "Familial Bony Dystrophy with Multiple Exostoses," *Radiology*, XXIV (1935): 623–625.
- "Amoebic Hepatitis," *J. Egypt. Med. Ass.*, XVIII (1935): 783–791.
- (with S. E. Harris) "Pneumococcus Meningitis Following Tonsillectomy and Terminating in Recovery," *Lancet*, CCXXX (1936): 143–144.
- (with E. W. Dennis) "An Outbreak of Epidemic Jaundice at Hamet, Lebanon," *Transactions of the Royal Society of Tropical Medicine and Hygiene*, XXXVII (1938): 186–196.
- (with W. Shehadi) "Duodenal Ulcer Syndrome Caused by Ankylostomiasis: Report of Twenty-Five Cases with Gastric Acidity and Roentgenological Studies," *Amer. J. Roentgenol*, XLIX (1943): 39–48, 129.
- "The Armenian National Sanatorium Azouneyeh, Lebanon," *Al Kulliyah* (1947).

Department of Neurology

Rahme, Edmond

- (with D. Green) "The Incidence of Subdural Hematoma in Adolescence and Adulthood," *J. Amer. Med. Association*, CLXXIII (1960).
- (M. W. Van Allen) "Lymphosacomatous Infiltration of the Cauda Equina," *Arch. Neurol.* (Chic), VII (1962): 476–481.

Sabra, Fuad A.; head of Neurology and chairman of the Department of Medicine

- (with H. Zellweger, and Y. Green) "The Clinical Diagnosis of Inclusion Body Encephalitis" (Dawson), *Helv. Paediat. Axta.*, XIII (1958): 81–87.
- "Observations on One Hundred Cases of Cerebral Angiomas," *J. Amer. Med. Association*, CLXX (1959): 1522–1524.
- (with H. A. Reimann) "Hereditary Spastic Paraplegia (Primary) Lateral Sclerosis. A Report of Three Cases in a Family," *M. E. Med. J.*, I (1962): 75–78.

- (with L. Ghandur-Mnaymneh) "Clinical Pathological Conference," *Lebanese Medical Journal*, XVII (1964): 429–440.
- (with M. Salam) "Pyogenic Infections of the Central Nervous System,"in Tinsley Harrison, ed., *Principles of Internal Medicine*, 5th ed. (New York: McGraw-Hill Book Co., 1964), 1168–1174.

Shorey, William D.

- "Localization of Intra-Cranial Tumors," *Lebanese Medical Journal*, VI (1953): 208–210.
- "Traumatic Aneurysm, a Case Report," *Leb J. Med.*, VI (1953): 49–54.

Department of Nutrition

McLaren, Donald; chairman

- *Malnutrition and the Eye* (New York and London: Academic Press, 1963).
- "A Study of the Factors Underlying the Special Incidence of Keratomalacia in Oriya Children in the Phulbani and Ganjam Districts of Orissa, India," *Journal of Tropical Medicine*, II (1956): 135–140.
- "Progressive Myopia in a Man of 60," letter to *British Medical Journal*, II (1957): 1192.
- "Chronic Protein Deficiency and Some Congenital Abnormalities of the Eye of the Rat," *Proceedings of the Nutrition Society*, XVI (1957): 23–24.
- "Congenital Abnormalities of the Eye of the Albino Rat Produced by Protein Deficiency," *Proceedings of the Fourth International Congress of Nutrition*, Paris (1957): 159–160.
- (with W. J. Darby) "Nutrition in Indonesia," *World Health Organization Restricted Circulation Report*, SEA/Nut./4 (1957).
- (with K. Bagchi) "Some Biochemical, Histological, and Clinical Effects of Malnutrition on the Eyes of Experimental Animals," *Proceedings of the Nutrition Society*, XVII (1958): 19.
- "Malnutrition and the Eye," *World Health Organization Technical Report Series*, no. 149 (1958): 32–35x.
- "Important Role of Malnutrition in Eye Disease," *East African Medical Journal*, XXXV (1958): 281–282.
- *"Complicaciones Oculars de la Malnutriticion Proteica,"* *Boletin de la Oficina Sanitaria Panamericana*, XLVI (March 1959).
- "Growth and Water Content of the Eyeball of the Albino Rat in Protein Deficiency," *British Journal of Nutrition*, XII (1958): 254–259.
- "Involvement of the Eye in Protein Malnutrition," *Bulletin of the World Health Organization*, XIX (1958): 303–313.
- "Cataract: a Biochemical Problem," letter to *Lancet*, I (1958): 1132.

- "The Pathogenesis of Hypovitaminosis A," *Federation Proceedings*, XVII (1958): 136.
- "Eye Diseases in African Children," letter to *British Journal of Ophthalmology*, XLIII (1959): 62.
- "The Eye and Related Glands of the Rat and Pig in Protein Deficiency," *British Journal of Ophthalmology*, XLIII (1959): 78–87.
- "Influence of Protein Deficiency and Sex on the Development of Ocular Lesions and Survival Time of the Vitamin A-Deficient Rat," *British Journal of Ophthalmology*, XLIII (1959): 234–241.
- "Urinary Excretion of Vitamin A in Pregnancy," *Proceedings of the Nutrition Society*, XVIII (1959): 30.
- "Records of Birth Weight and Prematurity in the Wasukuma of Lake Province, Tanganyika," *Transactions of the Royal Society of Tropical Medicine and Hygiene*, LIII (1960): 173–178.
- "Malnutrition and the Eye," *East African Medical Journal*, XXXVII (1960): 298–299.
- "The Crystalline Lens in Human and Experimental Malnutrition," *Proceedings of the Nutrition Society*, XIX (1960): 78.
- "Malnutrition and Eye Disease in Tanganyika," *Proceedings of the Nutrition Society*, XIX (1960): 89.
- "The Role of Malnutrition in Eye Disease. Results of Surveys in Lake and Central Provinces, Tanganyika," *East African Medical Journal*, XXXVII (1960): 321–331.
- "Kaposi's Sarcoma of the Eyelids of an African Child," *Archives of Ophthalmology*, LXIII (1960): 859–861.
- "Nutrition and Eye Disease in East Africa," Journal of Tropical Medicine and Hygiene, LXIII (1960): 101–121.
- "Visual Aquity Surveys," letter to *British Medical Journal*, II (1960): 308.
- (with W. J. Darby, W. J. McGanity, D. Paton, A. Z. Alemu, and A. M. Medhen) "Bitot's Spots and Vitamin A Deficiency," *Public Health Reports*, LXXV (1960): 738–743.
- "The Pattern of Early Growth in Sukumaland, Tanganyika," *Journal of Pediatrics*, LVI (1960): 803–813.
- (with D. Paton) "Bitot's Spots," *American Journal of Ophthalmology*, L (1960): 568–574.
- "Ocular Manifestations of Human Vitamin B Complex Deficiency," *Proceedings of the Fifth International Congress of Nutrition*, Washington (1960).
- "Malnutrition and Eye Disease in Two Bantu Tribes in East Africa," *Annales del Instituto Barraquer*, I (1960): 471.
- "Sources of Carotene and Vitamin A in Lake Province, Tanganyika," *Acta Tropica*, XVIII (1961): 79.
- "Ocular Lesions in Kwashirkor," letter to *British Medical Journal*, I (1961): 424.
- "The Effect of Malnutrition on the Eye, with Special Reference to Work with Experimental Animals," *World Review of Nutrition and Dietetics*, II (1961): 27.
- "Central American and East African Onchocerciasis Compared," *East African Medical Journal*, XXXVIII (1961): 193.

- "Nutritional Blindness," *Res Medicae*, II (1961): 38–43.
- "Nutritional Blindness," Transactions of the First Congress of the Asia Pacific Academy of Ophthalmology, (1961): 80–89.
- "The Refraction of Indian School Children: A Comparison of Data from East Africa and India," *British Journal of Ophthalmology*, XLV (1961): 604–613.
- (with M. J. Shaw and K. R. Dally) "Eye Disease in Leprosy Patients. A Study in Central Tanganyika," *International Journal of Leprosy*, XXIX (1961): 20–28.
- (with W. W. C. Read) "An Unusual Major Fatty Acid Component in Human Depot Fat," *Nature*, CXCII (1961): 265.
- (with P. G. Ward) "Malarial Infection of the Placenta and Fetal Nutrition," *East African Medical Journal*, XXXIX (1962): 182–189.
- (with W. W. C. Read) "Fatty Acid Composition of Adipose Tissue: A Study in Three Races in East Africa," *Clinical Science*, XXIII (1962): 247–250.
- "Xerophthalmia," American Journal of Clinical Nutrition, XI (1962): 603–609.
- "Ataxic Neurological Syndrome," letter to *British Medical Journal*, I (1963): 258.
- (with C. W. Woodruff, G. R. Barnley, J. T. Holland, D. E. Jones, and A. W. R. McCrae) "Onchocerciasis and the Eye in Western Uganda," *Transactions of the Royal Society of Tropical Medicine and Hygiene* (1963): 50–63.
- (with W. W. Johnstone) "Refraction Anomalies in Tanganyikan Children," *British Journal of Ophthalmology*, XLVII (1963): 95–108.
- "Nutritional Factors in Urinary Lithiasis," *East African Medical Journal*, XL (1963): 178–185.
- "World Hunger, Some Misconceptions," *Lancet*, II (1963): 86–87.
- "Bitot's Spots: A Review of Their Significance after 100 Years," *British Medical Journal*, II (1963): 926.
- "Nutritional Disease and the Eye," *Borden's Review of Nutrition Research*, XXV (1964): 1–16.
- "Vitamin A," letter to *Nutrition Reviews*, XXII (1964): 30.
- (with C. Ammoun, G. Houry, and I. Foster) "The Socio-Economic Background of Marasmus in Lebanon," *Lebanese Medical Journal*, XVII (1964): 85–96.
- (with C. Ammoun, G. Houry, and I. Foster) "Coronary Heart Disease in Lebanon, a Public Health Problem," *Lebanese Medical Journal*, XVII (1964): 15–22.
- (with A. H. Halasa) "The Refractive State of Malnourished Children," *Archives of Ophthalmology*, LXXI (1964): 827–831.
- "Biochemical Changes in Human Xerophthalmia," *American Journal of Clinical Nutrition*, XIV (1964): 241.
- "Xerophthalmia: A Neglected Problem," *Nutrition Reviews*, XXII (1964): 289–291.
- (with A. H. Halasa) "The Ocular Manifestations of Nutritional Disease," *Postgraduate Medical Journal*, XL (1964): 711–716.

- (with H. A. P. C. Oomen and H. Escapini) "Epidemiology and Public Health Aspects of Hypovitaminosis A, A Global Survey on Xerophthalmia," *Tropical and Geographical Medicine*, XVI (1964): 271–315.
- (with E. Shirajian, M. Tchalian, and G. Houry) "Xerophthalmia in Jordan," *American Journal of Clinical Nutrition*, XVII (1965): 117–130.
- (with M. Tchalian and Z. Ajans) "Biochemical and Hematologic Changes in the Vitamin A-Deficient Rat," *American Journal of Clinical Nutrition*, XVII (1965): 131–138.
- (with W. Kamel and N. Ayyoub) "Plasma Amino Acids and the Detection of Protein Malnutrition," *American Journal of Clinical Nutrition*, XVII (1965): 152–157.
- (with Z. A. Ajans and Z. Awdeh) "The Composition of Human Adipose Tissue, with Special Reference to Site and Age Differences," *American Journal of Clinical Nutrition*, XVII (1965): 171–176.
- "Vitamin A and Protein Relationships," letter to *Transactions of the Royal Society of Tropical Medicine and Hygiene*, LIX (1965): 103.
- "Biochemical Changes in Human Xerophthalmia," *Revue Médicale du Moyen Orient*, XXII (1965): 112–120.
- (with H. A. P. C. Oomen and H. Escapini) "Ocular Manifestations of Human Vitamin A Deficiency in Man," *Bulletin of the World Health Organization*, XXXIV (1966): 357–361.
- "Present Knowledge of the Role of Vitamin A in Health and Disease," *Transactions of the Royal Society of Tropical Medicine and Hygiene*, LX (1966): 436–462.
- "A Fresh Look at Protein-Calorie Malnutrition," *Lancet*, II (1966): 485–488.
- "The Prevention of Xerophthalmia," *Pre-School Child Malnutrition*, Publication 1282, Washington, DC: National Academy of Science–National Research Council (1966): 96–101.
- (with P. Asfar) "Vitamin A in Serum and Liver in Relation to Serum Proteins and Liver Pathology in Kwashiorkor and Marasmus," *American Journal of Clinical Nutrition*, XVIII (1966): 304.
- "Nutritional Status of People in Isolated Areas of Puerto Rico," letter to *American Journal of Clinical Nutrition*, XVIII (1966): 467.
- "An Early Account of Infant Feeding Practices and Malnutrition in East Africa," *Journal of Tropical Medicine*, XII (1966): 50–52.
- "Protein Calorie Malnutrition," letter to *Lancet*, II (1966): 592.
- "Trends in Tropical Child Health," *Journal of Tropical Medicine*, XII (1966): 84–85.
- "A Simple Scoring System for Classifying the Severe Form of Protein Calorie Malnutrition of Early Childhood," *Lancet* (1967): 533–535.
- "Patients Who Reside in Common Lodging-Houses," *British Medical Journal*, I (1967): 497.
- "Study of Vitamin A Deficiency in Young Children," in *U.S. Department of Health Education and Welfare Public Health Service* (March 1967): 213–221.
- "Brain Drain," *Science*, CLVI (1967): 1497.

- "Nutritional Disorders of the Eye," in A. Sorsby, ed., *Modern Trends in Ophthalmology*, 4th ed. (London: Butterworths,1967), 130–144.
- *Study of Vitamin A Deficiency in Young Children*, report to the Republic of Nigeria Nutrition Survey Interdepartmental Committee on Nutrition for National Development (Washington, DC: US Government Printing Office, 1967).
- (with H. A. P. C. Omen and H. Escapini) *"Encusta mundial sobre la xeroftalmia," Reimpreso del Bolrtin de la Oficina Sanitaria Panamericana*, LXII (1967).
- "Population, Food and Disease in the Near East," in Fuad Sarruf and Suha Tamin, eds., *A.U.B. Festival Book (Festschrift)* (Beirut: American University of Beirut Centennial Publications, 1967), 185–219.

Department of Ophthalmology and Ear, Nose, and Throat
[prior to division into two separate departments]

Abu-Jaudeh, Caezar

- "A Giant Phinolith," *Laryngoscope*, LXI (1951): 271.
- "The Occurrence of Inclusion Bodies in the Epithelium of the Nasal and Urethral Mucous Membranes of Trachomatous Patients: A Preliminary Report," *Am. J. Ophthal.*, XXXV (1953): 947–956.
- "Clinical Significance of Hoarseness," *Lebanese Medical Journal*, VII (1954): 126–131.
- "Simple Method to Reduce Bleeding during Tonsillectomy," *Laryngoscope*, LXVII (1957): 93–95.
- "Melkerson's Syndrome," *Ann. Otol.* (St. Louis), LXIX (1960): 989–996.
- "Orbital Complications in Otolaryngology," *Ann. Otol.* (St. Louis), LXXI (1962): 934–945.
- (with A. Diab) "Aureomycin in Trachoma," *Am. J. Ophthal.*, XXXV (1952): 1187–1190.
- (with A. Diab) "Sulfonamides in Trachoma," *Am. J. Ophthal.*, XXXV (1952): 1339–1342.
- (with A. Diab) "Respiration Distress in Infancy," *Am. Otol.* (St. Louis), LXVI (1956):198–207.

Baghdassarian, Aram S.

- (with J. Mamo) "Beket's Disease. A Report of 28 Cases," *Archives of Ophthalmology*, LXXI (1964): 4–14.

Diab, Alfred E.; chairman

- "Clinical Application of Bronchoscopy," *Lebanese Medical Journal*, III (1950): 89–96.
- (with C. S. Matta) "Surgical Correction of Cicatricial Entropion and Trichiasis. A Report of 244 Cases," *Am. J. Ophthal.*, XXXIX (1955): 355–358.

Halasa, Adnan H.

- "Corneal Infection due to B-Pyocyaneus. A Case Report," *Lebanese Medical Journal*, XVI (1962?): 21–28.
- (with M. F. Armaly) "The Effect of External Compression of the Eye on Intraoccular Pressure. I. Its Variation with Magnitude of Compression and with Age," *Invest. Ophthal.*, II (1963): 591.
- (with M. F. Armaly) "The Effect of External Compression of the Eye on Intraoccular Pressure. II. Recovery: Tonographic Changes and the Influence of Pharmacologic Agents," *Invest. Ophthal.*, II (1963): 599.
- "Varicose Veins of the Eyelids," *Archives of Ophthalmology*, LXXI (1964): 176–179.
- "Amyloid Disease of Eyelid Conjunctiva," *Archives of Ophthalmology* (in press).
- "Medical Treatment of Malignant Glaucoma," *American Journal of Ophthalmology* (in press).

Department of Otolaryngology

Abu-Jaudeh, Caezar N.

- "A Giant Phinolith," *Laryngoscope*, LXI (1951): 271.
- "The Occurrence of Inclusion Bodies in the Epithelium of the Nasal and Urethral Mucous Membranes of Trachomatous Patients: A Preliminary Report," *American Journal of Ophthalmology*, XXXV (1953): 947–956.
- "Clinical Significance of Hoarseness," *Lebanese Medical Journal*, VII (1954): 126–131.
- "A Sample Method to Reduce Bleeding during Tonsillectomy," *Laryngoscope*, LXVII (1957): 93–95.
- "Melkerson's Syndrome," *Ann Otol.* (St. Louis), LXIX (1960): 989–996.
- "Orbital Complications in Otolaryngology," *Ann Otol.* (St. Louis), LXXI (1962): 934–945.
- (with A. Diab) "Aureomycin in Trachoma," *American Journal of Ophthalmology*, XXXV (1952): 1187–1190.
- (with A. Diab) "The Sulfonamides in Trachoma," *American Journal of Ophthalmology*, XXXV (1952): 1339–1342.
- (with A. Diab) "Respiration Distress in Infancy," *Ann Otol.*, (St. Louis), LXVI (1957): 198–207.

Baghdassarian, Aram S.

- (with J. Mamo) "Becket's Disease. A Report of 28 Cases," *Archives of Ophthalmology*, LXXI (1964): 4–14.

Diab, Alfred E.

- "Clinical Application of Bronchoscopy," *Lebanese Medical Journal*, III (1950): 89–96.
- (with C. N. Abu-Jaudeh) "The Sulfonamides in Trachoma," *American Journal of Ophthalmology*, XXXV (1952): 1339–1342.
- (with C. N. Abu-Jaudeh) "Aureomycin in Trachoma," *American Journal of Ophthalmology*, XXXV (1952): 1187–1190.
- (with C. S. Matta) "Surgical Correction of Cicatricial Entropion and Trichiasis, A Report of 224 Cases," *American Journal of Ophthalmology*, XXXIX (1955): 555–558.
- (with C. N. Abu-Jaudeh) "Respiration Distress in Infancy," *Ann Otol.*, (St. Louis), LXVI (1957): 198–207.

Karam, Farid K.

- "Otosclerosis in Lebanon," *Lebanese Medical Journal*, XVI (1963): 210–215.
- (with S. Salman) "Meningioma of the Middle Ear," *Arch. Otolaryng.*, LXXX (August 1964).

Mamo, Jubran G.

- (with A. S. Baghdassarian) "Becket's Disease–A Report of 28 Cases," *Archives of Ophthalmology*, LXXI (1964): 4–14.

Matta, Camille S.

- (with A. Diab) "Surgical Correction of Cicatricial Entropion and Trichiasis. A Report of 224 Cases," *American Journal of Ophthalmology*, XXXIX (1955): 555–558.

Department of Pathology

Ghandur-Mnamymneh, Latifeh

- (with J. L. Wilson, S. S. Saleh, H. D. Yacoubian, and I. K. Dagher) "Absorption of Blood from the Pericardium," *J. Thorac. Cardiovasc. Surg.*, XLIV (1962): 785–792, 810–812.
- (with W. Mnaymneh, and H. R. Dudley) "Giant Cell Tumor of Bone," *J. Bone. JT. Surg.*, XLVI–A (1962): 63–75.
- (with M. S. Slim, H. D. Yacoubian, J. L. Wilson, and G. A. Rubeiz) "Successful Reimplantation of the Canine Lungs," *Surg.*, LV (1964): 676–683.
- (with M. A. Shamma'a) "Clinico-Pathological Conference," *Lebanese Medical Journal*, XVII (1964): 141–152.

- (with J. Moadie) "Clinico-Pathological Conference," *Lebanese Medical Journal*, XVII (1964): 289–298.
- (with S. Firzli) "Clinico-Pathological Conference," *Lebanese Medical Journal*, XVII (1964): 349–358.
- "Liver Cell Carcinoma Causing Extra-Hepatic Obstructive Jaundice," *Lebanese Medical Journal* (1964): 333–337.
- (with F. Sabra) "Clinico-Pathological Conference," *Lebanese Medical Journal*, XVII (1964): 429–440.
- (with J. Moadie) "Clinico-Pathological Conference," *M. E. Med. J.*, II (1965): 43–55.
- (with E. R. Harrison, R. M. Dajani, and T. Nassar) "The Utilization of Ethanol. III. Liver Changes Induced by Alcohol," *J. Nutr.*, LXXXVI (1965): 29–36.

Sahyoun, Philip F.; chairman

- (with M. Bodansky and M. E. Blish) "Experimental Fetal Nephritis," *Proceedings of the Society for Experimental Biology and Medicine*, XXXI (1938): 7–13. [**Nassar comment:** this article was not available from the Saab Medical Library.]
- (with H. G. Dorman) "Identification and Significance of Spirochetes in the Placenta," *Am. J. Obs. Gyn.*, XXXIII (1937): 954–967.
- (with A. Oppenheimer) "Some Fresh Aspects of Appendicitis. A Joint Roentgenological and Histopathological Study," *Amer. J. Roentgenol*, LXI (1939): 188–197.
- "The Differentiation between Spirochetes and Spirochete-like Structures in the Placenta," *Amer. J. Path.*, XV (1939): 455–466.
- (W. M. Bickers and A. Saadeh) "Granulosa Cell Tumor of the Ovary," LXXIV (1947): 509–512.
- (with W. M. Bickers, and M. Massie) "Vaginal Cervical Smears in the Diagnosis of Uterine Cancer," *Virginia Medical Monthly*, LXXV (1948): 568–574.
- (with R. B. Smith, J. K. Finnegan, P. S. Larson, M. L. Dreyfuss, and H. B. Haag) "Toxicologic Studies on Zinc and Disodium Ethylene Bidithiocarbomates," *Journal of Pharmacology and Experimental Therapy*, CIX (1955): 159–166.
- (with H. A. Riemann and H. T. Chaglassian) "Primary Amyloidosis Relationship to Secondary Amyloidosis, and Report of a Case," *Arch. Int. Med.*, XCIII (1954): 673–686.
- (with H. A. Reiman, J. Moadie', and S. Smerdjian) "Periodic Peritonitis. Heredity and Pathology. Report of 72 Cases," *J. Amer. Med. Association*, CLIV (1954): 1254–1259.

Sproul, Edith E.; 1946–1949, 1956–1957

- (with J. J. McDonald, and R. Lattes) "Non-Chromaffin Paraganglioma of Carotid Body and Orbit. Report of a Case," *Ann. Surg.*, CXXXIX (1954): 382–384.
- "Occult Metastases in the Spine," *Proc. VIIth M.E. M.A.* (1956): 1M–8M.

Tuqan, Nimr, A. F.

- (with R. Blount, E. Goyette, A. D. Wright, and R. Murray) "Atherosclerosis and Hypertension" (A 55-6HN 88241), C.P.C., *Proc. M.E.M.A.* (1956).
- (with P. H. Wood, P. D. White, R. Maingot, R. Brock,and G. Saleeby) "Hypertension and Atherosclerosis" (A 55-42 HN 5142), C.P.C., *Proc. VIIth M.E.M.A.*(1957).
- (with A. McGehee Harvey, C. E. Dent, H. A. Reimann, I. Roache, J. Stahl, and W. Shehadi) "Bilateral Pneumonia with Jaundice, Atherosclerosis, and Hypertension" (A 56-4 HN 100 843), C.P.C., *Proc. VIIIth M.E.M.A.* (1956).
- (with S. Firtzli) "Clinico-Pathological Conference," *Lebanese Medical Journal*, XI (1958): 45–54.
- (with Sir H. Ogilivie) "Congenital Cystic Lymphangioma of the Greater Curvature of the Omentum," C.P.C., *Lebanese Medical Journal*, XI (1958): 134–145.
- "Adenoma of the Tracheo Bronchial Tree. A Clinico-Pathological Study," *Lebanese Medical Journal*, XI (1958): 175–191.
- "Periodic Disease: A Clinico-Pathological Study," *Ann. Inter. Med.*, XLIX (1958): 885–899.
- "Liver Infarction and Subacute Bacterial Endocarditis following Biliary Surgery," C.P.C., *Lebanese Medical Journal*, XI (1958): 215–228.
- (with R. A. Tabbara) "Clinical-Pathological Conference, Transposition of the Great Vessel. Inter-Auricular and Inter-Ventricular Septal Defects," *Lebanese Medical Journal*, XI (1958): 317–332.
- (M. Katrib, F. S. Haddad, and S. Haddad) "Primary Carcinoma of the Ureter," *A. R. Orient Hosp.*, XI (1958): 51–64.
- "Disseminated Lupus Erythematosus. (Anemia and Joint Pains)," C.P.C., *Lebanese Medical Journal*, XII (1959): 85–96.
- (with G. Dragatsi) "Clinico-Pathological Conference. Epigastric Pain, Melena, and Gastric Filling Defect," *Lebanese Medical Journal*, XII (1959): 210–218.
- (with F. S. Haddad, R. Cattel, J. Merrvill, D. Browne, G. Fanconi, and G. W. Saleeby) "Intestinal Obstruction," C.P.C., *Lebanese Medical Journal*, XII (1959): 309–327.
- (with G. W. Saleeby) "Primary Reticulum Cell Sarcoma of the Spleen," *Radiology*, LXXII (1959): 868– 873.
- "Two Types of Cirrhoses," C.P.C., *Lebanese Medical Journal*, XII (1960): 240–253.
- (with C. W. M. Adams) "Elastic Degeneration as Source of Lipids in the Early Lesion of Atherosclerosis," *J. Path. Bact.*, LXXXII (1961): 131–139.
- "Linitis Plastica of Inflammatory Nature—a Pitfall in the Diagnosis of Gastric Carcinoma," *Lebanese Medical Journal*, XIV (1961): 300–307.
- (with F. S. Haddad) "Renal Lipomatosis. (Mass in Right Loin and Non-Functioning Right Kidney), C.P.C., *Lebanese Medical Journal*, XVI (1961): 314–323.
- (with C. W. M. Adams) "The Histochemical Demonstration of Protease by a Gelatin-Silver Film Substrate," *Journal of Histochemistry and Cytochemistry*, IX (1961): 469–472.

- (with C. W. M. Adams) "Histochemistry of Myelin-I Proteins and Lipid-Protein Complexes," *J. Neurochem.*, VI (1961): 327–333.
- (with C. W. M. Adams) "Histochemistry of Myelin. II. Proteins, Lipid Proteins Dissociation and Proteinase Activity in Wallerian Degeneration," *J. Neurochem.*, VI (1961): 334–341.
- (with D. Ingvar, F. S. Haddad, E. I. Shwayri, S. Cronquist, and F. Sabra) "Clinic-Pathological Conference. Brain Abscess and Uremia," *Middle East Medical Journal* (1952): 79–90.
- "The Range of Reliability of the Liver Biopsy," *M. E. Med. J.* (1962): 25–56.
- (with F. Hanger) "Jaundice and Uremia," C.P.C., *M. E. Med. J.* (1962): 271–282.
- "Physicians of Confuseland," *J. Amer. Med. Ass.* (April 14, 1962): 218, 220.
- "Annular Stricture of the Esophagus Distal to Congenital Trachea Esophageal Fistula," *Surgery*, LII (1962): 394–395.
- (with Shafik Haddad) "Diabetes, Mass, and Shock," C.P.C., *M. E. Med. J.*, I (1962): 179–190.
- (with C. W. M. Adams) "Histochemistry of Demyelination," *Ann. Histochem*, VIII (1963): 215–222.
- (with S. Firzli) "Veno-Occlusive Disease of the Liver," C.P.C., *Lebanese Medical Journal*, XVII (1963): 65–74.
- "Giant Cell Carcinoma of the Lung," *Lebanese Medical Journal*, XVII (1964): 407–412.
- "The Lobular Pattern of the Skin, an Approach to the Histological Interpretation of Cutaneous Lesions," *Brit. J. Derm.*, LXXVI (1964): 322–329.
- (with S. Firzli) "Clinico-Pathological Conference," *Lebanese Medical Journal* (1964): 351–358.
- "The Stroma, Its Descriptive and Applied Anatomy," *Guy's Hosp. Rep.*, CXIII (1964): 111–121.
- "Primary Dissecting Aneurysm of the Renal Artery," *J. Path. Bact.*, LXXXIX (1965): 369–370.
- "Some Observations on Congenital Diaphragmatic Hernias," *J. Path. Bact.*, LXXXIX (1965): 370–372.
- Safeguards against Pathological Pathology of Thyroid Neoplasms," *Lebanese Medical Journal*, XVIII, sup. 5 (1965): 419–459.

Department of Pediatrics

Firzli, Salim. (see also, papers of the Department of Pathology)

- (H. Zellweger and L. Giaccai) "Gargoylism and Morquio's Disease," *Amer. J. Dis. Child.* LXXXIV (1952): 321–435.
- Anemies Hypoplastiques de L'enfance Rev. Med. De Moy. Or. XIII (1955): 258–261.

- (with F. Hamawi and H. Zellweger) "Malignant Tumors in Early Life," *Leb. Med. J.*, VIII (1955): 13–36.
- (with H. Zellweger) "Hodgkin's Disease in Children, a Clinical Study," *Ann. Paediat. Basel*, CXXXIX (1957): 381–385.
- (with N. A. Tuqan) "Seoto-Meningitis in Infancy," C.P.C., *Leb. Med. J.*, XI (1958): 45–54.
- "*Crise aplastique dans la thalasemie*," *Rev. Med. Moy. Or.*, XVII (1960): 74–82.
- "Splenectomy in Thalassemia," *Turk. J. Pediat.*, IV (1962): 39–44.
- (with L. Ghandour-Mnaymneh) "Clinical-Pathological Conference," *Lebanese Medical Journal*, XVII (1964): 348–358.
- (with M. S. Slim, and R. E. Melhim) "Staphylococcic Pneumonia in Infants under the Age of Six Months," *Dis. Chest*, XLVII (April 1965).

Idriss, Hassan

- (with R. Kegel and H. Nachman) "Treatment of Intussusceptions in Infants," *Rev. Med. Liban.*, I (1948): 242–246.
- (with L. Giaccai) "Osteomeylitis due to Salmonella Infection," *J. Ped.*, XLI, 1952, 73–78.
- (with H. Zelleger) La regulation nerveuse de l'homeostase et sa pathologie. J. Swisse Med., LXXXIX (1959): 958–964.
- (with H. Zellweger) "Encephalopathy in Salmonella Infections," *Amer. J. Dis. Child.*, LXLIX (1960): 770–777.
- (with M. Salam) "Cystic Fibrosis in the Pancreas in the Middle East. Report on Five Cases," *Lebanese Medical Journal*, XV (1962): 61–74.
- (with M. S. Slim and J Bitar) Hypertrophy of the Pyloric Mucosa. A Rare Cause of Congenital Pyloric Stenosis," *Amer. J. Dis. Child.*, CVII (1964): 636–639.
- (with M. Salam) "Infantile Amaurotic and Family Idiocy and Gargoylism in Siblings," *Pediatrics*, XXXIV (1964): 658–666.
- (R. Kegel and H. Nachman) "The Treatment of Acute Intussusceptions in Infants," *Rev. Med. Lib.*, I (1948): 242–246.

Nachman, Henry; chairman

- (with S. S. Najjar) "The Kocher-Debre'-Semelaigne Syndrome," *Journal of Pediatrics*, LXVI (1965): 901–908.

Najjar, Samir; chairman

- (with Z. Ajans) "Diabetes Insipides following Clinical Mumps," *Amer. J. Dis. Child.*, CII (1961): 865–867.

- "Respiratory Manifestations in Infants with Hypothyroidism," *Rcch. Dis. Childh.*, XXXVII (1962): 603–605. [**Nassar comment:** This article is another example of important clinical research with observations that may shed light on the problem of infant crib death and its relationship to infant hypothyroidism (cretinism included) as being the cause of crib death. It is not well known that hypothyroidism below one year of age (eight infants were studied), with its depression of respiratory center function, promotes the occurrence of sleep apnea and its pathophysiological morbidity and mortality, which, if not diagnosed and treated early, may lead to crib death. In addition, the myxedema fluid may hamper the bellows action of the thorax. Further clinical research based on the article of Dr. Samir Najjar awaits to amplify the relationship of hypothyroidism and apnea and crib death so that treatment and prevention of the latter becomes routine practice.]

- (with S. Nassif) "Congestive Heart Failure in Infancy due to Hypothyroidism," *Acta Paediat.* (Uppsala) (1962): 319–326. [**Nassar comment:** It is well documented that congestive heart failure may cause Cheyne-Stokes disordered breathing, and this clinical search report documents a case of hypothyroidism in a nineteen-day old female infant with normal delivery at term, who developed secondary congestive heart failure post-delivery. Again here is a possible relationship to crib death that may occur secondary to respiratory depression complicating the seriousness of symptoms of heart failure and cardiac arrhythmias. Sudden infant deaths (SIDs) was noted to occur most commonly up to six months following delivery, and it occurs during infants' sleep. Because death is sudden, it is postulated that it may be due to an arrhythmic event secondary to a prolonged Q-T interval. According to reports in the literature, prolonged Q-T interval is caused by a mutation of either of two genes—SCN 5 or KVLT—at birth.*Prolonged Q-T interval may predispose to torsades de pointes. Additionally presence of congestive heart per se, is a risk for dangerous arrhythmias. (*)L. J. Gula and coworkers, "Clinical Relevance of Arrhythmias during Sleep: Guidance for Clinicians," *Heart* 90(3) (March 2004): 352-374.]

- (with C. Woodruff) "Some Observations on Goiter in Lebanon," *American Journal of Clinical Nutrition*, XIII (1963): 46–54.

- (Pendred's Syndrome in Two Families Living in an Endemic Goiter Area," *B. M. J.*, II (1963): 31–33.

- (with K. Younoszai and V. Der Kaloustian) "Hypothyroidism in Children. A Review of 47 Cases," *Lebanese Medical Journal*, XVI:181–196.

- (with A. Jarrah) "Pigmentation in Addison's Disease," *Amer. J. Dis. Child.*, CVII (1964):198–201.

- "Hypothyroidism in Children from an Endemic Goiter Area," *J. Pediat.*, LXIV (1964): 372–380.

Nassif, Sami I.; cardiology–subspecialty pediatric cardiology, cited in the Department of Pediatrics

- (with S. S. Najjar) "Congestive Heart Failure in Infancy due to Hypothyroidism," *Acta Peadiat.* (Uppsala), LII (1963): 319–325. Refer to comment under the Department of Pediatrics with coauthor Dr. Samir Najjar.

Salam-Adams, Maria

- (with H. Zellweger and L. Giaccai) "Craniostenosis with Multiple Epiphyseal Displasias and Congenital Dislocation of Hip Joints," *Helv. Paediat. Acta.*, VII (1952): 185–192.
- (with F. Sabra) "Pyogenic Infection of the Central Nervous System," in T. Harrison, ed., *Principles of Internal Medicine*, 5th ed. (New York: McGraw Hill Co., 1965), 1168–1174.
- (with J. Rubeiz, and R. D. Adams) "Clinical Neurology and Classification of Muscle Disease," in T. R. Harrison, ed., *Principles of Internal Medicine*, 5th ed. (New York: McGraw Hill Co., 1965), 1264–1268.
- "Pediatric Neurology—an Emerging Subspecialty of Medicine in the U.S.A. with a Brief Commentary on Its Potential Development in the Middle East," *Leb. Med. J.*, XVIII (1965): 495–510.
- (with F. Khoury) "The Enigma of the Eccentric Chromosome, the Aberrant Chromosome and the Maring of the Brain," *Lebanese Medical Journal*, XIX (1966): 3.
- (with H. Ayoub, and A. Zareir) "Report on the International Congress on the Scientific Study of Mental Retardation," *Lebanese Medical Journal* XVIII, (1946): 209–222.
- (with H. Idriss) "Infantile Amaurotic Ffamily Idiocy and Gargoylism in Siblings," *Pediatrics*, XXXIV (1964): 658–666.
- (with W. Shanklin) "A Comparison of the Histochemistry of the Central Cortex from Siblings with Gargoylism and Tay-Sachs Disease," *Acta Neuroveg* (Wien), XXV (1963): 297–309.
- (with H. Idriss) "Cystic Fibrosis of the Pancreas in the Middle East," *Lebanese Medical Journal*, XV (1962): 61–74.
- "Phenylketonuria in a Child from the Middle East," *Amer. J. Dis. Child.*, CV (1963): 102–103.
- (with W. M. Shanklin, and M. Issidorides) "Histochemistry of the Cerebral Cortex from a Case of Familial Amaurotic Idiocy," *J. Neuropath. Exp. Neuro.*, XXI (1962) : 284–293.
- (with D. D. Matson) "Brain Abscess in Congenital Heart Disease," *Ped.*, XXVII (1961): 772–789.
- "Cystic Fibrosis of the Pancreas in an Oriental Child," *Ann. Paediat.* (Basel), CXC (1958): 252– 255.
- (with H. Zellweger) "Hurler's Disease and Neurofibromatosis in a Family," *Helv. Paedit. Acta*, XII (1957): 633–642.

- (with H. Zellweger) "Neurofibromatosis," *Rev. Med. Moy. Or.*, XVI (1957): 289-384.
- (with E. Rizk and H. Zellweger) "Intestinal Parasitism in Lebanon. A Statistical Analysis of 1,000 Children," *Ann. Paediat.* (Basel), CLXXXV (1955): 310.
- (with L. Giaccai and H. Zellweger) "Cleidocranial Dysostosis with Osteopetrosis Acta," *Radiol.* (Stockh.), XLI (1954): 417–424.
- (with L. Giaccai and H. Zellweger) Dyostose cleoidocraniene osteopetrose et oligophrenie Journees Medicales de Beyrouth. II (1952): 297.

Woodruff, Calvin, W.; faculty, chairman

- "Vitamin Deficiency (Survey) in Control of Malnutrition in Man" (New York: American Public Health Association, 1960): 53–56.
- (with K. Hoermann) "Nutrition of Infants and Preschool Children in Ethiopia," *Pub. Hlth. Rep.—Nutrition*, LXXV (1960): 724–730.
- "Folic Acid Deficiency in Control of Malnutrition in Man" (New York: Public Health Association, 1960): 64–65.
- "Protein Requirements of Full Term Infants: Report to the Council on Food and Nutrition," *J. Amer. Med. Ass.*, CLXXXV (1961): 114–118.
- "The Utilization of Iron Administered Orally," *Ped.*, XXVII (1962): 149–198.
- (with K Hoermann) "Blood Proteins in Residents of Egypt: Differences in Capillary Samples as Observed in Permanent and Transient Residents," *Arch. Environm. HLTH.*, II (1961): 673–678.
- (with G. Barmley, J. Holland, D. James, A. McCrea, and D. S. MacLaren) "Onchocerciasis and the Eye in Western Uganda," *Trans. Roy. Soc. Trop. Med. and Hyg.*, LVII (1953): 50–63.
- (with S. S. Najjar) "Some Observations on Goiter in Lebanon," *Am. J. Clin. Nut.* (1963): 46–54.

Zellweger, Hans U.; 1951–1959, chairman

- (with L. Giaccai, and Maria Salam) "Craniostenosis with Multiple Epiphyseal Displasias and Congenital Dislocation of Hip Joints," *Helv. Paediat. Acta*, VII (1952): 185–192.
- (with L. Giaccai, and M. Salam) "*Dysostose Cleidocranienne, osteopetrose et oligophrenie,*" J. *Medicales de Beyrouth*, II (1952): 297–299.
- (with L. Giaccai, and S. Firzli) "Gargoylism and Morquio's Disease," *Amer. J. Dis. Child.*, LXXXIV (1952): 421–434.
- Betrachtungen zum problem der kinderkrampfe. *Disch. Med. Wschr.*, LXXVIII (1953): 1253–1259.
- (with I. Giaccai) Contibuto ala conscenza della sindrome di Fanconi-de toni. ATTI XVII *Congr. Radiologia Medica* (1952).
- "Clinical Aspects of Poliomyelitis," *Lebanese Medical Journal*, VI (1953): 153–168.

- (with M. Ghandour) "Modern Trends in Poliomyelitis with Special Consideration of the Outbreak in Lebanon in 1952," *Lebanese Medical Journal*, VI (1953): 1–19.
- (with L. Giaccai) Die infantile cortical hyperostose und lbre differential diagnose. *Mod. Probl. Padiat.* I, fasc. 58 (1954): 806–812.
- (with L. Giaccai and M. Salam) "Cleidocranial Dysostosis with Osteopetrosis Acta," *Radiol.* (Stockh.), XLI (1954): 417–424.
- (with W. H. Adolph) Vitamin und vitamin-krankheiten. Handbook der inneren inern Medizin 4, Aufl. Bd. VI 5, (1954): 687–826.
- (with F. S. Farah and A. N. Acra) "Secondary Renal Hyperchloremic Acidosis Complicated by Other Tubular Functions," *Helv. Paediat. Acta.*, X (1955): 324–341.
- (with A. J. Dark and G. I. Abu Haidar) "Glycogen Storage Disease of Skeletal Muscle. Report of Two cases and Review of the Literature," *Pediatrics*, XV (1955): 715–732.
- (with S. Firzli and F. Hammani) "Malignant Tumors in Early Life," *Lebanese Medical Journal*, VIII (1955): 13–36.
- Malformations medullaris chey l'enfant. Encyclopedie Me'dico-Chirurgical 4100 D 10, (1955), 1–3.
- Traumatismes obstetricaux de la moelle e'piniere 4100 D 10, (1955), 1–2.
- (with E. Rizk and M. Salam) "Intestinal Parasitism in Lebanon," *Ann. Paediat.*, CLXXXV (1955): 310–319.
- Glykogenspeicherkrankheiten. Dtch. Med. Wschr. LXXXI (1956): 1907–1914.
- (with S. Firzli) Zur Differential diagnose maligner lymphoma in kindsalter. Eine Statistisch –klinische studie mit kasuitischen beitragen. Helv. Paediat. Acta, XI (1956): 1–23.
- (with R. E. Melhim and H. Doumanian) "Hurler's Disease in Infancy and Early Childhood," *Helv. Paediat. Acta.*, XII (1957): 606–632.
- (with P. S. Mugerditchian) "Congenital Broncho-Esophgeal Fistula in an Adult," *Lebanese Medical Journal*, IX (1956): 225–233.
- (with S. Firzli) "Hodgkin's Disease in Children, a Clinical Study," *Ann. Paediat.* (Basel), CLXXXIX (1957): 381–385.
- (with M. Salam) "Hurler's Disease and Neurofibromatosis in a Family," *Helv. Paediat. Acta*, XII (1957): 633–642.
- "Problems of Childhood Tubersulopsis," *Lebanese Medical Journal*, X (1957): 68–86.
- (with M. Salam) "Neurofibromatose," *Rev. Med. Moy. Or.*, XIV (1957): 384.
- (with F. Sabra, and Y. Green) "The Clinical Diagnosis of Inclusion Body Encephalitis" (Dawson), *Helv. Paediat. Acta*, XIII (1958): 81–87.
- "Convulsions in Childhood," *Ann. Paediat.*, CXC (1958): 257–277.
- "Vaccinations against Poliomyelitis and Its Indications in Lebanon," *Lebanese Medical Journal*, XII (1959): 42–52.
- (with H. Idriss) La regulation de nerveuse de l'homeostase et sa pathologie. Schweiz. Med. Wschr., LXXXIX (1959): 958–964.

Department of Pharmacology

Fawaz, George A.; professor and chairman

[**Nassar comment:** George A Fawaz, PhD, MD, chairman of the department, is one of the pillars of AUB.]

- (Farah Alfred) "The Determination of the Minimal Lethal Dose and the Average Rate of Uptake of G-Strophanthin and Digitoxin in the Heart Lung Preparation of the Dog," *J. Pharm. Esp. Therap.* (abstract), vol. 86, no. 2 (February 1946): 101–112.
- Uber die Solanin. Dissertation, Universität Graz, 1937.
- Lieb H & Zacherl MK: Zur Kenntnis der Phosphatide und Cerebroside. Biochem Z (1937): 293–121.
- Zeile K & Fawaz G: Synthese der naturlichen-Kreatin-Phosphorsaure. Z Physiol Chem 1938 256 193.
- Fawaz G & Zeile K: Synthese einiger organischer Phosphorsaure-Verbindungen. Z Physiol Chem 1940 263 175.
- Zeile K, Fawaz G & Ellis W: Uber die Reduktion der Katalase. Z Physiol Chem 1940 263 181
- (with A. Farah) "Digitoxin-Binding Power of Serum and Other Soluble Tissue Proteins of the Rabbit," *J Pharmacol & Exp Therap* (1944): 80 193.
- (with K. Seraidarian) "Phosphoglycocyamine," *J Biol Chem* (1946): 165 97.
- (withvK. Seraidarian) "The Structure of Adenosine Triphosphate," *J Am Chem Soc* (1947): 69 966.
- (with F. Bergmann) "Condensation of l,l-Diaryl-Ethylenes with Maleic Anhydride," *J Am Chem Soc* (1947): 69 1773.
- (with L. F. Fieser, et al.) "Naphthoquinone Antimalarials," *J Am Chem Soc*, I (1948): 70 3151.
- (with L. F. Fieser, et al.) "Naphthoquinone Antimalarials," *J Am Chem Soc*, X (1948): 70 3174.
- (with L. F. Fieser and M. G. Ettinger) "Distribution of Naphthoquinone Antimalarials between Organic Solvents and Aqueous Buffers," *J Am Chem Soc* (1948): 70 3228.
- "The Role of the Liver in the Tolerance to Morphine in the Rat," *Proc Soc Exp Biol & Med* (1948): 68 262.
- (with L. F. Fieser) "A New Synthesis of Lapinone," *J Am Chem Soc* (1950): 72 996.
- (with E. N. Fawaz) "Mechanism of Action of Mercurial Diuretics," *Proc Soc Exp Biol & Med* (1951): 77 239.
- "The Mechanism by Which Dibenamine Protects Animals against Cardiac Arrhythmias," *Brit J Pharmacol* (1951): 6 492. [**Nassar comment:** My research on whether dibenamine is available for clinical use to prevent cardiac arrhythmias during

anesthesia in humans did not show any results; although in this experimental work by Dr. Fawaz, dibenamine was supplied by Smith Kline and French Laboratories, in Philadelphia, PA, and Sterling–Winthrop Research Institute, Rensselaer, NY. Dr. Fawaz reported that dibenamine does protect the intact dog's heart from arrhythmias under cyclopropane or chloroform anesthesia from adrenaline but not in the isolated heart, but protects the isolated dog's heart from *l*–noradrenaline, and from iosoprenaline.]

- (with Farid S. Haddad) "The Effect of Lapinone on P. vivax Infection in Man," *Am J Trop Med* (1951): 31 569.
- (with H. Meyer) "Rat Poison from White Squill," *Brit J Pharmacol* (1953): 8 440.
- (with E. S. Hawa) "The Phosphocreatine Content of Mammalian Cardiac Muscle," *Proc Soc Exp Biol & Med* (1953): 84 277.
- (with E. N. Fawaz) "Effect of Metabolites on the Accumulation of Citric Acid in Fluoracetate-Poisoned Rats," *Proc Soc Exp Biol & Med* (1953): 84 680.
- (with E. N. Fawaz) "Mechanism of Action of Mercurial Diuretics," *Proc Soc Exp Biol & Med*, II (1954): 87 30.
- "Effect of Quinidine, Procaine Amide and Mersalyl on the Lethal Dose of Ouabain in the Dog Heart-Lung Preparation," *Proc Soc Exp Biol & Med* (1955): 88 654.
- Die Wirkung von Fluoressigsaure auf Leistung und Stoffwechsel des Hertzlungenpraparates des Hundes. Arch Exper Path u Pharmakol (1956): 288·377.
- (with E. N. Fawaz and B. Tutunji) "Effect of Metabolites on the Accumulation of Citrate in the Fluorocitrate-Poisoned Rat," *Proc Soc Exp Biol & Med* (1956): 92 311.
- (with E. S. Hawa and B. Tutunji) "The Effect of Dinitrophenol, Hypoxemia and Ischemia on the Phosphorus Compounds of the Dog Heart," *Brit J Pharmacol* (1957): 12 270. [**Nassar comment:** The experiments were on the isolated dog heart under the following conditions: (1) The effect of dinitrophenol, which acts directly on the myocardium, causes marked increase in oxidatrive metabolism (metabolic rate), which also results in heart failure associated with decrease of phosphor creatine content in the muscle, but no change in adenosins triphosphate. (2) The same effect result is demonstrated under hypoxemia. Similarly with ligation of coronary arteries.]
- (with B. Tutunji) "The Mechanism of Dinitrophenol Heart Failure," *Brit J Pharmacol* (1957): 12 273. [**Nassar comment:** Dinitrophenol infused in the heart-lung preparation was shown to increase cardiac metabolic rate and in larger doses of dinitrophenol, hypoxemia results, which were found to be an important factor in the resultant heart failure. Phosphocreatin was decreased in the absence of heart failure in smaller dose of dinitrophenol.]
- (with B. Tutunji and E. N. Fawaz) "Effect of Malonate on Performance and Metabolism of the Isolated Dog Heart," *Proc Soc Exp Biol & Med* (1958): 97 770.
- (with B. Tutunji) "Ouabain-Induced Ventricular Tachycardia and Its Effect on the Performance and Metabolism of the Dog Heart," *Brit J Pharmacol* (1959): 14 355. [**Nassar comment:** Determination of oxygen consumption of the dog heart-lung preparation was made at constant pressure work. Following induction of atrial

tachycardia by direct atrial stimulation, oxygen consumption of the myocardium increased greater than control level and much greater with toxic doses of ouabain-induced ventricular tachycardia but not with therapeutic doses of ouabain, suggesting increased desaturation in coronary sinus blood with toxic doses. It was interesting to note that, during the drug-induced ventricular tachycardia, there was no decrease in phosphocreatine content nor in the nucleotide phosphorus content of the myocardium in the absence of hypoxia.]

- (with B. Tutunji) "The Effect of Adrenaline and Noradrenaline on the Metabolism and Performance of the Isolated Dog Heart," *Brit J Pharmacol* (1960): 15 389.
- "The Effect of Mephentermine on Isolated Dog Hearts, Normal and Pretreated with Reserpine," *Brit J Pharmacol* (1961): 16 309.
- (with E. N. Fawaz) "Inhibition of Glycolysis in Rat Skeletal Muscle by Malonate," *Biochem J* (1962): 83 438.
- (with E. N. Fawaz, G. Fawaz, andK. von Dahl)" Enzymatic Estimation of Phosphocreatine," *Proc Soc Exp Biol & Med* (1962): 109 38.
- (with E. Manoukian) "Steady-State Level of Phosphocreatine in the Heart," *Circ Res* (1962): 11 115.
- (with E. N. and K. von Dahl) The Effect of Insulin on Some Triphosphopyridine Nucleotide-Employing Enzymes," *Enzym Biol Clin* (1962): 2 73.
- (with J. Simaan) "Cardiac Noradrenaline Stores," *Brit J Pharmacol* (1963): 20 569.
- (with K. von Dahl) "The Enzymatic Estimation of Ammonia in Tissues and Body Fluids," *Leb Med J* (1963): 16 169.
- "Cardiovascular Pharmacology," *Ann Rev Pharm* (1963): 3 57.
- (with J. Simaan) "The Chronotropic actions of Guanethidine and Reserpine on the Isolated Dog Heart," *Arch Exp Path u Phamak* (1964): 247 452.
- (with J. Simaan) "On the Mechanism of the Pressor Action of Tyramine," *Arch Exp Path u Pharmak* (1964): 247 456.
- (with J. Simaan) "Mechanism of Tachyphylacxis to Tyramine and Mephenterrnine," *Arch Exp Path u Pharmak* (1965): 250 247.
- (with J. Simaan) "The Tachyphylaxis Caused by Mephentermine and Tyramine," *Brit J Phannacol* (1965): 24 526.
- "The Mechanism by Which Noradrenaline Restores the Pressor Action of Indirectly Acting Sympathomimetic Amines in Reserpinized Dogs," *Brit J Pharmacol* (1966): 26 282.
- (with E. N. Fawaz and L. Roth) "The Enzymatic Estimation of Inorganic Phosphate," *Biochem Z* (1966): 344 212.
- "Effect of Reserpine and Pronethalol on the Therapeutic and Toxic Actions of Digitalis in the Dog Heart-Lung Preparation," *Brit J Pharmacol* (1967): 29 302.
- (with J. Simaan) "Effects of Dipyridamole on the Dog Heart-Lung Preparation," *Cardiovasc Res* (1968): 2 68.

- (with J. Simaan) "The mechanical Efficiency of the Starling Heart-Lung Preparation." *Pflügers Arch* (1968): 302 123.
- (with J. and M. Slim) "The Effect of Chronic Cardiac Sympathectomy on the Therapeutic and Toxic Actions of Digitalis in the Dog Heart-Lung Preparation," *Arch Pharmak u Exp Path* (1968): 261 212.
- (with E. Manoukian) "The Enzymatic Microestimation of Urea," *Z klin Chem u klin Biochem* (1969): 7 32.
- (with E. Manoukian) "The Enzymatic Estimation of Free and Combined Adenine," *Z klin Chem u klin Biochem* (1970): 8 599.
- (with J. Simaan) "Effect of Endogenous Catecholamines and Norepinephrine on the Performance of the Isolated Canine Heart," *Arch f Exp Pharmak* (1971): 268 17.
- (with E. Fawaz) "Phosphate Compound Analyses," in A. Schwartz, *Methods in Pharmacology* (New York: Appleton-Century-Crofts, 1971), 1 515.
- (with J. Simaan) "Is Pressure Work of the Isolated Canine Heart Dependent on Release of Catecholamines?" *Arch f Pharmak* (1971): 270 136.
- (with J. Simaan and S. Jarawan) "The Effect of Ouabain-Induced Contractility on Myocardial Oxygen Consumption," *Arch f Pharmak* (1971): 271 249–61.
- (with E. Manoukian) "The Enzymatic Microestimation of Inosine, Adenosine and Inosinic Acid," *Z Physiol Chem* (1971): 352 1631.
- (with J. Simaan) "The Metabolic Effect of Noradrenaline on the Isolated Canine Heart after Blockade of the Chronotropic Action by Veratramine," *Arch f Pharmak* (1973): 277 199.
- (with J. Simaan) "The Effect of Theophylline Alone and in Combination with Ouabain on the Isolated Dog Heart," *Arch f Pharmak* (1973): 278 45.
- (with J. Simaan) "Myocardial Oxygen Consumption in Isovolumic Hearts with Varying Cardiac Outputs," *Cardiovasc Res* (1974): 8 763.
- (with J. Simaan) "Dissociation between the Chronotropic and Inotropic Actions of Glucagon," *Naunyn-Schmiedebergs Arch f Pharmak* (1974): 283 293.
- (with J. Simaan) "The Cardiodynamic and Metabolic Effects of Glucagon," *Naunyn-Schmiedebergs Arch f Pharmak* (1976): 294 277.
- (with J. Simaan) "The Cardiodynamic and Metabolic Effects of Verapamil on the Isolated Dog Heart," *Naunyn-Schmiedebergs Arch f Pharmak* (1979): 310 139.
- (with J. Simaan) "The Metabolic Effects of Carbochromen and Propranolol on Isolated Dog Heart," *Naunyn-Schmiedebergs Arch f Pharmak* (1980): 314 171.
- (with E. Fawaz, E. Manougian, and J. Simaan) "Uric Acid Formation in the Dog Lung," *Mol & Cell Biochem* (1982): 43 111.
- (with J. Simaan and K. Jabbur) "Comparison of the Cardiodynamic and Metabolic Effects of Dobutamine with Those of Norepinephrine and Dopamine in the Dog Isolated Heart," *Naunyn-Schmiedebergs Arch f Pharmak* (1988): 338 174.
- "Sixty Years of Cardiovascular Physiology and Pharmacology with Special Reference to Cardio-Active Steroids and Sympathomimetic Amines (monograph in preparation).

- (with E. Manougian) "Steady-State of Phosphocreatine in the Heart," *Circulat. Res.*, XI (1962): 115–118.
- (with E. Manougian and E. Fawaz) "Glycolysis in Dog Skeletal Muscle," *Biochem. Z*, CCCXXXVII (1963): 195–201.
- Bibliography of nonscientific papers, some of which have not been published:
- Introduction to "Allemagne 70," *Orient Suppl* (January 25, 1970).
- Dr. Philip Sahyun, 1978.
- Mittagessen speech, January 16, 1981.
- *Gaudeamus igitur juvenes dum sumus* [Let us be merry while we are young]. Toubib (1981): 33.
  - ≠ "Whither AUB? An Excursion through the Campus Lasting Five-Score Years and Ten," *MEJ Anesth* (1983): 7(1, 2) 9–19.
  - ≠ "A Rare Bird of Passage Alights on the AUB cCmpus and Stays for Three Years. Otto Krayer (1899–1982) as I knew him," *Medicus* (1983): 14(1) 10-5.
  - ≠ "The Physician in Politics," *Medicus* (1983): 14(2) 10-4.
  - ≠ "The Cultured Physician," (commencement speech June 27, 1983). *Leb Med J* (1983): 33 249-60.
- Mittagessen speech May 24, 1984. (The author writes on November 9, 1994: "The speech is in German. It is good that not everybody knows German. I do not want our people in the ME to read it.")
- Afif Mufarrij (medical commencement June 25, 1984).
  - ≠ "When the Great Meet: Frederick II of Prussia and Voltaire," *Medicus* (1984): 15 9-11.
  - ≠ "Reflections on Grace Dodge Guthrie's Book: A Legacy to Lebanon," 1985. [The author writes on November 9, 1994: "The AUB Information Office sent this paper to Mr. Muhammad àliy alruzz who sent it to Mr. R. G. Berry, the editor of the AUB Newsletter which appears in the US, with a great complimentary letter to the author; the editor interpreted the paper as a 'sectarian discourse' and did not publish it."]
  - ≠ "Uber das Negative." A student paper c. 1985.
  - ≠ "Cornerstones: Edwin St. John Ward, BA, MD, FACS, DSc," *Medicus* (1986): 16 10-6.
  - ≠ "Cornerstones: SE Kerr," Published in Medicus.
  - ≠ "Reminiscences of an Alumnus: AUB in the Early Thirties—Its Golden Age," *SCAN* (1987): 5(1) 6-14.
  - ≠ "The American University of Beirut—Yesterday, Today and Tomorrow," (May 1987). [The author writes on November 9, 1994: "This paper should not be read by Americans. Although it was written in 1987, I subscribe to everything written in it."]
  - ≠ "I Remember Suleiman Daud Deeb," *Al-Kulliyah* (Autumn 1988):15-7.

- ≠ "Elias J. Corey: The greatest organic chemist of all times?" (May 28, 1991). [The author writes on November 9, 1994: "It summarizes some of the things I had made."]
- ≠ "The Influence of University Education on the Inborn Traits of Human Nature," *Sci-Quest* (1993): 3(1) 31-2.
- ≠ "The Life of a Scientist: Werner Heisenberg, the Scientist and the Man," *Sci-Quest* (1994): 4(1) 16-24.
- ≠ "Denkstruktur," *Sci-Quest* (1994): 4(2) 16-23.
- • On the "expiration" date of drugs. [The author writes on November 9, 1994: "This is a good article. Your brother Fuad as one of the editors of the *Leb Med J* sent it to the journal for publication, but it was not published. I think the editor-in-chief, whoever he was, was afraid of the drug companies. You see we are governed not only by politicians but also by Big Industry—I am attempting now to have it published in Germany in one form or another. Actually, it should be published in the USA! Everything that is written there is true. What a pity that we dump into the sea billions worth of drugs when poor people are left untreated. I sent the article, a few weeks ago, to an important man in the German Pharmacological Society. Let us see what he has to say." November 9, 1994.]
- ≠ "Habib Kurani," (June 18, 1994). [The author writes on November 9, 1994: "His memorial took place 11 years after his death. Habib's wife and daughter came to Beirut for this purpose. It ends by a word from Grace Dodge which she asked me to read in her behalf."]
- ≠ "Dr. Musa Ghantus, as I Knew Him."
- ≠ "Dr. Mustafa Khalidy, a Doctor for the People."
- ≠ "Tamer Nassar, of the Histology Department."

Department of Physiology

Badeer, Henry S.; chairman

[**Nassar comment:** Truly a remarkable and excellent physiologist, his experiments on the etiology or pathophysiology on the occurrence of ventricular fibrillation following the occlusion of the coronary artery in dogs' hearts and review of the literature on the subject is of great importance. Among the concepts worked on, it appeared that trigger zones between an infracted cardiac muscle area and ischemic area nearby or noninfracted muscle is not a direct cause for ventricular fibrillation, similarly in dogs' hearts following hypoxic hypoxia. However, it appeared from his experiments that extrusion of intracellular potassium into the coronary circulation does have significance on the production of ventricular fibrillation and is corrected with infusion of glucose with insuli, similarly with the effect of magnesium infusions. It is of interest to note that, from our clinical observations (Dr. Richard Stock and I, and colleagues) and electrocardiographic recordings on patients with myocardial infarcts, the occurrence of ventricular ectopic systole on the T wave produced ventricular fibrillation. Refer to chapter 4 and my work at the Monitoring Unit.]

- "The Neuro-Endocrine Control of Renal Excretion of Water," *Leb. Med. J.*, I (1948): 123–131.
- "Influence of Temperature on S-A Rate of Dog's Heart in Denervated Heart-Lung Preparation," *Amer. J. Physiol.*, CLXVII (1951): 76–80.
- "Influence of Oxygen on Hypothermic Cardiac Standstill in the Heart-Lung Preparation," *Circulat. Res.*, III (1955): 28–31.
- "Role of Hypoxia in Hypothermic Cardiac Arrest in the Heart-Lung Preparation," *Amer. J. Physiol.*, CLXXXIII (1955): 119–120.
- (with A. K. Khachadurian) "Effect of Hypothermia on Oxygen Consumption and Energy Utilization of Heart," *Circulat. Res.*, IV (1956): 523–526.
- "Effect of Hypothermia on Aerobic Energy Utilization of Heart," in *Abstracts of Communications*, XXth International Physiological Congress, Brussels, Belgium (1956): 52.
- (contributor to) "Table 264, Heart Rates," in W. S. Spector, ed., *Handbook of Biological Data* (Ohio: Wright AV Development Center, Wright-Patterson Air Force Base, 1956), 277.
- "Ventricular Fibrillation 10 Hypothermia," *J. Thorac. Surg.*, XXXV (1958): 265–273.
- (with A. K. Khachadurian) "Role of Bradycardia and Cold Per Se in Increasing Mechanical Efficiency of Hypothermic Heart," *Amer. J. Physiol.*, CXCII (1958): 331–334.
- (with S. M. Horvath) "Role of Acute Myocardial Hypoxia and Ischemic-Nonischemic Boundaries in Ventricular Fibrillation," *Amer. Heart J.*, LVIII (1959): 706–714.
- "Table 47. Effect of Temperature on Heart Rate: Vertebrates (Parts II and III)," in D. S. Dittmer and R. M. Grebe, eds. *Handbook of Circulation* (Ohio: Aerospace Medical Laboratory, Wright-Patterson Air Force Base, 1959), 96–98.
- (with A. K. Khachadurian) "Effect of Tolbutamide on Glucose Utilization by the Denervated Heart-Lung Preparation," *Metabolism*, IX (1960): 890–896.
- "Effect of Heart Size on the Oxygen Uptake of the Myocardium," *Amer. Heart J.*, LX (1960): 948–954.
- (with A. K. Khachadurian and J. D. Karam) "Effect of Tolbutamide on Glucose and Oxygen Uptake and Coronary Flow on the Isolated Dog Heart," *Arch. Int. Pharmacodyn.*, CXXXII (1961): 42–48.
- "Importance of Oxygen Differentials in the Etiology of Ventricular Fibrillation after Ligation of the Coronary Artery," *Amer. Heart J.*, LXIII (1962): 374–380.
- "Role of the Pericardium in the Application of the Starling Mechanism to Unanesthetized Animals," *Amer. Heart J.*, LXIII (1962): 427–428.
- "Work Capacity of the Hypothermic Heart," *Amer. Heart J.*, LXIII (1962): 839–840. [**Nassar comment:** This Annotation by Dr. H. S. Badeer proposed a clear definition of the "work capacity" of the hypothermic heart that avoided the confusing definitions

in the physiology literature, such as minute work capacity, stroke work capacity, and total work capacity of the isolated heart. From a clinical standpoint, the hypothermic heart has a reduced minute work capacity and it is recommended that it should not be overloaded by output or arterial pressure.]

- "A Plea for Standardization of Definitions in Cardiovascular Functions," *Amer. Heart J.*, LXIV (1962): 432–433.
- "Editorial—Current Concepts on the Pathogenesis of Ventricular Fibrillation Soon after Coronary Occlusion," *Amer. J. Cardiol.*, XI (1963): 709–713.
- "Physiologic Basis for the Normally Low Oxygen Content of Coronary Venous Blood," *Amer. Heart J.*, LXV (1963): 844–846.
- "Relative Influence of Heart Rate and Arterial Pressure on Myocardial Oxygen Uptake," *Acta Cardiol.* (Brux.), XVIII (1963): 356–365.
- "Clinical Progress—The Stimulus to Hypertrophy of the Myocardium," *Circulation*, XXX (1964): 128–136.
- "Editorial—Biological Significance of Cardiac Hypertrophy," *Amer. J. Cardiol.*, XIV (1964): 133–138.
- (with S. H. Ghalib) "Heart Weight to Body Weight Ratio in the Dog," *Leb. Med. J.*, XVII (1964): 327–331.
- "Influence of Cooling the Heart on Reactive Hyperemia of the Coronary Bed in the Heart-Lung Preparation," *Circulat. Res.*, XVI (1965): 19–25.
- (with K. Abu Feisal) "Effect of Atrial and Ventricular Tachycardia on Cardiac Oxygen Consumption," *Circulat. Res.*, XVII (1965): 330–335.

Jabbur, Suhayl J.

- (with R. P. Bircher) "Toxic Effects of Cardiac Glycosides and Antidotal Effects of Different Compounds in the Cat," *Fed. Proc.*, XVI (1957): 282.
- (with A. L. Towe) "Blocking and Excitation of Cuneate Neurons by Sensori-Motor Cortical Stimulation in the Cat," *Fed. Proc.*, XVIII (1959): 73.
- (with A. L. Towe) "Cortical Potential Evoked by Isolated Pyramidal Tract Stimulation," *Fed. Proc.*, XVIII (1959): 160.
- (with O. A. Smith and R. F. Rushmer) "Effects of Diencephalic Stimulation on Cardiovascular Responses in Close-Chested Dogs," *Fed. Proc.*, XVIII (1959): 147.
- (with O. A. Smith Jr. and R. F. Rushmer) "Effects of Diencephalic Stimulation and Ablation on Cardiovascular Responses in the Chronic Preparation," *Int. Congr. Physiol.*, XXI (Buenos Aires, 1959): 257.
- (with A. L. Towe) "Antidromic Cortical Response to Isolated Pyramidal Tract Stimulation in the Cat," *Science*, CXXIX (1959): 1676–1678.
- (with D. A. Smith Jr. and R. F. Rushmer) "Lesions of Hypothalamic Cardiovascular Regulatory Areas and the Resulting Degeneration," *VIIth Int. Anat. Congr.* (1960): 280.

- (with D. A. Smith Jr., R. F. Rushmer, and E. P. Lasher) "Role of Hypothalamic Structures in Cardiac Control," *Physiol. Rev.*, XL, suppl. 4, pt. 2 (1960): 136–141.
- (with A. L. Towe) "Effects of Pyramidal Tract Activity on Dorsal Column Nuclei," *Science*, CXXXII (1960): 547–548.
- (with A. L. Towe) "The Influence of the Cerebral Cortex on the Dorsal Column Nuclei," in E. Florey, ed., *Nervous Inhibition, Proceedings of the Second Friday Harbor Symposium* (New York: Pergamon Press, 1961), 419–423.
- (with A. L. Towe) "Cortical Inhibition of Dorsal Column Nuclei of Cat," *J. Neurophysiol.*, XXIV (1961): 499–509.
- (with A. L. Towe) "Analysis of the Antidromic Cortical Response Following Stimulation of the Medullary Pyramids," *J. Physiol.* (Lond.), CLV (1951): 148–160.

Khuri, Raja N.

- (with D. L. Maude, I. Shehadeh, and A. K. Solomon) "Na and H20 Transport in Single Perfused Distal Tubules of Necturus Kidney," *Fed. Proc.*, XXIII (1964): 305.
- (with C. R. Merril) "Blood pH with and without a Liquid-Liquid Junction," *Phys. in Med. Biol.*, IX (1964): 541–550.
- "Glass Microelectrodes and Their Uses in Biological Systems," in George Eisenman, ed., *Glass Electrodes for Hydrogen and other Cations: Principles and Practice* (New York: Marcel Dekker, Inc., Fall 1965).

Department of Psychiatry

Drooby, Ala'uddin S.

- "Changing Child Rearing Patterns in the Middle Eastern Family," *Leb. Med. J.*, XIII (1960): 50–53.
- "The Psychiatrist's Role in the Management of Mentally Retarded Children's Parents," *Leb. Med. J.*, XV (1962): 100–105.
- "A Reliable Truce with Enuresis," *Diseases of the Nervous System*, XXV (1964): 97–100.

Garabed, Aivazian

- "Medico-Legal Aspects of Psychiatry in Lebanon with a Review of Some Justice Cases," *Leb Med. J.*, VI (1952): 37–48.

Racy, John Cecil

- "What Is Psychosomatic Medicine," *Leb Med J* (1961): 14 pp 372, 492.
- "Psychosomatic Dentistry," *Rev Dent Lib* (1962): 12 53.

- "Family Interactions in Health and Disease," *Leb Med J* (1962): 15 247.
- "Of Matter and Mind," *Leb Med J* (1962): 15 297.
- (with E. J. Lynn) "The Rsolution of Pathological Grief after Electroconvulsive Therapy," *Journal of Nervous & Mental Disease* (February 1969): 148(2): 165–169.
- "How Does a Group Grow?" *Arner J Nurs.* (November 1969) (11): 2396–2400.
- (with H. Katchadourian) "The Diagnostic Distribution of Treated Psychiatric Illness in Lebanon," *Brit J Psych.* (November 1969): 115(528): 1309–1322.
- "Death in an Arab Culture," *Ann NY Acad Sci.*(December 19, 1969): 164(3): 871–880.
- "Psychiatry in the Arab East," *Acta Psych Scand* (1970) sup. 211: 1–171.
- "Ten Misuses of Sex," *Med Asp Hum Sex.* (February 5, 1971): 136–145.
- (with R. H. Goldstein, D. M. Dressler, R. A. Ciottone, and J. R. Willis) "What Benefits Patients? An Inquiry into the Opinions of Psychiatric Inpatients and Their Residents," *Psych Quart.* (1972) 46(1): 49–80.
- (with H. Penn, L. Lapham, M. Mandel, and J. Sandt) "Catatonic Behavior, Viral Encephalopathy, and Death. The Problem of Fatal Catatonia," *Arch Gen Psych.* (December 1972): 27(6): 758–761.
- "Islam," in R. H. Cox, ed., *Religious Systems and Psychotherapy* (Springfield: CC Thomas, 1973), 156–166.
- (with A. Klepfisz) "Homicide and LSD," *JAMA* (January 1973): 22 223(4): 429–430.
- "How the 'Work Ethics' Influences Sexuality," *Med Asp Hum Sex.* (April 1974): 8(4) 84.
- "A Foreign Graduate with US Training Reimmigrates to the United States," *Archives of Surgery* (September 1974): 109(3): 365–366.
- (with R. H. Goldstein) "Residents' Perceptions of Inpatient Psychiatric Care," *Comprehensive Psychiatry* (March–April 1975): 16(2): 171–177.
- (with J. Ciccone) "Psychotic Depression and Hallucinations," *Comprehensive Psychiatry* (May–Inn 1975): 16(3): 233–236.
- "Psychiatrists as Administrators: Problems of Leadership and the Exercise of Power," *Hospital & Community Psychiatry* (August 1975): 26(8): 528–529.
- "Psychiatry in the Arab East," in L. C. Brown and N. Itzkowitz, eds., *Psychological Dimensions of Near Eastern Studies* (Princeton: Darwin Press, 1977), 279–329.
- "How Sexual Relationships Mirror the Total Relationship," *Med Asp Hum Sex* (August 1977): 11(8) 98.
- "Psychiatric History: Potential for Abuse" [letter], *American Journal of Psychiatry* (November 1978): 135(11): 1437–1438.
- "Stress and Human Disease. An Overview and Background," *Arizona Medicine* (May 1980): 37(5): 352–354.
- (with E. A. Ward-Racy) "Tinnitus in Imipramine Therapy," *Am J Psych* (July 1980): 137(7): 854–855.
- "Somatization in Saudi Women: a Therapeutic Challenge," *Brit J Psych.* (September 1980): 137: 212–216.

- (with S. Nasr and J. A. Flaherty) "Psychiatric Effects of the Civil War in Lebanon," *Psych J Univ Ottawa* (December 1983): 8(4): 208–212.
- "The Family and Chronic Disease," *Ariz Med.* (December 1983): 40(12): 854–857.
- "Psychological Adaptations to Amputations: an Overview," *Orthotics & Prosthet* (1985): 38(3) 46–50.
- (with L. E. Beutler) "A View from the Podium," *Intern J Eclect Psych* (1986) 5(5).
- "Psychological Aspects of Amputation," in J. M. Malone and W. S. Moore, eds., *Lower Extremity Amputation* (Phil: WB Saunders, 1989), 330–340.
- (with J. W. Smith and P. C. Ferry) "Tenure for a New Age. Ideas for the Turn of the Century" [editorial] [see comments], *Arch Int Med.* (May1989): 149(5):1001.
- "Professionalism: Sane and Insane" [editorial], *Journal of Clinical Psychiatry* (April 1990): 51(4):138–140.
- "Psychological Adaptation to Amputation," in J. H. Bowker and J. W. Michael, *Atlas of Limb Prosthetics: Surgical, Prosthetics, and Rehabilitation Principles*, 2nd ed. (St. Louis: Mosby, 1992), 707–716.
- "Limb Amputation," in F. S. Sierles, ed., *Behavioral Science for Medical Students* (Baltimore: Williams & Wilkins, 1993), 415–420.
- Not listed above are 10 book reviews, 14 brief communications, 11 abstracts and other publications, 70 presentations at major professional meetings (from 1973), and 168 lectures and media presentations (from 1973).

ROBERTSON, W. M. Ford

- "Some Problems Concerning the Approach to a Middle East Psychiatric Service," *Leb. Med. J.*, V (1952): 2–12.
- "The Concept of the Mental Hospital as a Therapeutic Community," *Leb. Med. J.*, VII (1954): 89–97.
- "Panel on Psychosomatic Medicine," *Proc. Vth M.E.M.A.* (1955): 544–557.

Department of Roentgenography

Giaccai, Leonardo M.

- (with H. Zellweger and M. Zabnienska) "Craniostenosis with Multiple Epiphyseal Displasias and Congenital Dislocation of Hip Joints," *Helv. Paediat. Acta*, VII (1952): 185–192.
- (with H. Zellweger and S. Firzli) "Gargoylism and Morquio's Disease," *Amer. J. Disc. Child.*, LXXXIV (1952): 421–435.
- (with H. Idriss) "Osteomyelitis due to Salmonella Infection," *J. Pediat.*, XLI (1952): 73–78.

- "Familial and Sporadic Neurogenic Acro-Osteolysis," *Acta Radiol.* (Stockh.), XXXVIII (1952): 17–29.
- (with H. Zellweger) "Contributo alla conoscenza della Syndrome di Fanconi – De Toni," *Atti SVII Congr. Radiologia Medica*, (1952).
- (with M. Salam and H. Zellweger) "Dysostose cleido-cranienne et osteopetrose et oligophrenie," *Journees Medicales de la Faculte Francaise de Medecine et de Pharmacie du Beyrouth*, II (1952): 297–299.
- "Acropachidermia con pachiperiostos," *Atti XVII Congr. Radiologia Medica*, (1952).
- (with U. Manjini) "Esistono nel quadro della syndrome pomboscia-talgica da ernia del disco disturbi del simpatico?" *Arch "Putti" Chir. Org. Movimento*, II (1952): 283–295.
- "Recent Advances in Radiotherapy," *Leb. Med. J.*, VI (1953): 196–203.
- (with M. Salam and H. Zellweger) "Cleidocranial Dysostosis with Osteopetrosis," *Acta Radiol.*, (Stockh.), XLI (1954): 417–424.
- (with H. Zellweger) "Die Infantilecortical hyperostose und ihre differential diagnose," *Moderne Probleme der Padratrie*, I, fasc.58 (1954): 806–812.
- "La diastematomyetie," *Rev. Med. Moy. Or.*, XI (1954): 359–364.
- "Concetti attuali sulla terapia del cancro della mammilla," *Nunt. Radiol. (Roma)*, XXII (1956): 70–78.
- "Il problema diagnostic et therapeutics del carcinoma *in situ* del lollo uterico," *Radiol. Med. (Torino)*, XLII (1956): 366–377.

Melhem, Rafic E. (1960–)

- (with H. Zellweger and H. Doumanian) "Hurler's Disease in Infancy and Early Childhood," *Helv. Paediat. Acta*, XII, fasc. 6 (1957): 606–632.
- (with J. Srouji and J. L. Wilson) "Hydatid Cyst of the Lung with Bronchographic Evaluation of Treatment by Internal Suture of the Pericyst," *J. Thorac. Surg.*, XXXV (1958): 779–794.
- (with N. K. Atallah) "Annular Pancreas in Infancy. Report of 3 Cases," *Amer. J. Roentgenol.*, XC (1963): 740–745.
- (with M. S. Slim) "Congenital Pulmonary Air Cysts—Successful Segmental Resection in 50-Day-Old Infant," *Arch Surg.*, LXXXVIII (1964): 923–926.
- (with J. J. Hajjar and N. Balassanian) "Histiocytosis X–A Report of 15 Cases in the Paediatric Age Group," *Brit. J. Radiol.*, XXXVII (1965): 898–904.
- (with S. Firzli and M. S. Slim) "Staphylococcic Pneumonia in Infants under the Age of Six Months," *Dis. Chest*, XLVII (1965): 6–13.

Saleeby, George W.

- (with A. Oppenheimer) "Proctography: Roentgenologic Studies of the Rectum and Sigmoid," *Surg. Gynec. Obstet.*, LXIX (1939): 83–93.

- "Cancer of the Tongue in Young Subjects with Report of a Case," *Amer. J. Cancer*, XXXVIII (1940): 257–262.
- (with P. H. Wood, P. D. White, R. Maingot, R. Brock, and N. A. Tuqan) "Hypertension and Atherosclerosis (A 55-42 HN 51413) C.P.C.," *Proc VIIth M.E.M.A.* (1957).
- (with F. S. Haddad, R. Cattell, J. Mervill, D. Brown, G. Fanconi, and N. A. Tuqan) "Urinary Obstruction (Intenstinal Obstruction), C.P.C.," *Leb. Med. J.*, XII (1959): 309–326.
- (with N. A. Tuqan) "Primary Reticulum Cell Sarcoma of the Spleen," *Radiology*, LXXII (1959): 868–871.

Shehadi, William H.

- "Primary Pyogenic Osteomyelitis of the Articular Processes of the Vertebrae," *J. Bone Jt. Surg.*, XXI (1939): 969–976.
- *Clinical Radiology of the Biliary Tree* (NY: Blakston, Division of McGraw Hill, 1963), 305.[**Nassar comment:** Dr. William H. Shehadi was a pioneer in the specialty of diagnostic radiology, especially prior to ultrasonography of liver-gallbladder-biliary tree scans, because he wrote the above clinical textbook, which in effect opened the development of clinical research in radiology.]

Department of Surgery

The honorable specialty of surgery rose into prominence at the end of the Christian Millennium, championed by Abul Quassim, Khalafi bin Abbas az Zahrawi (Albucasis 1013), who lived in the Versailles of Andalusia. Hemophilia as a sex-linked inheritance is accredited to his medical-surgical procedures that included his operative and clinical records. He illustratively described two hundred surgical instruments, many he designed himself.

—C. Elgood, *A Medical History of Persia and the Eastern Caliphate* (Cambridge 1957), quoted by Dr. Farid S. Haddad, *Leb. Med. J.* (1968): 67–80.

Azoury, Bahij; Department of Surgery, Division of Urology

- "Vesicovaginal Fistula," *Journal of Urology*, LXXV (1956): 75–78.
- "Anastomosis of Stenosed Uterine Cervix to Urinary Bladder," *Obstetrics and Gynecology*, XII (1958): 113–114.
- (with J. Moadié) "Schistosomiasis in Lebanon: A Report of the First Authentic Case," *Lebanese Medical Journal*, XIV (1961): 216–219.

Dagher, F. J.

[**Nassar comment:** Dr. F. J. Dagher is mentioned here to emphasize the clinical research that was instrumental by Dr. F. J. Dagher in performing the first kidney transplant operation for end-stage kidney disease in one twin from a donor brother with success at the AUB Medical Center Hospital in 1971, assisted by Drs. Kamal Hemady and Bahige Azoury from the Urology Division; a first surgical event in Lebanon and in the Middle East.]

Dagher, Ibrahim K.

- (with A. P. Hovnanian) "Intrabiliary Rupture of Hydatid Cyst of the Liver," *Ann. Surg.*, CXLI (1955): 263–267.
- (with J. J. McDonald) "Ankylosis of the Temporomandibular Joint," *Oral Surg.*, X (1957): 1145–1155.
- (with Clowes) "Failure of the Circulation III Acute Hypoxia," *Surg. Forum*, VII (1957): 197.
- (with F. A. Bashour) "Repeated Extraction of Needles from the Heart," *Leb. Med. J*, XI (1958): 157–166.
- (with others) "A Review of the Complications of Resection in the Treatment of Pulmonary Tuberculosis," *Surg, Gynee. Obstet.*, CIX (1959): 61–66.
- (with F. A. Bashour, J. Khalaf, and F. Fuleihan) "Right Aortie Arch: Report of Two Adult Cases," *Leb. Med. J.*, XII (1959): 75–84.
- "Pressure Membrane Oxygenator," *J. Thorac. Surg.*, XXXVII (1959): 100–107.
- (with H. G. Mishalani) "Mechanisms of Pulmonary Hypertension in Severe Hypoxia," *Proc. Xth. M.E.M.A.* (1960): 469–488.
- (with others) "Early Complications of Pulmonary Resection for Tuberculosis and Their Prevention," *Leb. Med. J.*, XIII (1960): 363–370.
- (with H. G. Mishalany and F. Simeone) "Mechanisms of Pulmonary Hypertension in Acute Hypoxia," *J. Thorac. Cardiovase. Surg.*, XLII (1961): 743–754.
- "Preliminary Report on Open-Heart Surgery," *Arab Med. J.* (1961): 22.
- "Surgical Care of the Wounds and of Injuries to the Blood Vessels," *M. E. Med. J.*, I (1962): 67–74.
- (with J. L. Wilson, S. S. Saleh, H. D. Yacoubian, and L. Ghandur-Mnaymneh) "The Absorption of Blood from the Pericardium," *J. Thorac. Cardiovase. Surg.*, XLIV (1962): 785–792, 810–812.
- (with G. A. Rubeiz, M. Nassar, S. Nassif, H. D. Yacoubian, R. A. Tabbara, and J. L. Wilson) "Open Intracardiac Repair of Tetralogy of Fallot," *Leb. Med. J.*, XVII (1964): 7–14.
- (with G. A. Rubeiz and M. Nassar) "Study of the Right Atrial Pressure Pulse in Functional Tricuspid Regurgitation and Normal Sinus Rhythm," *Circulation*, XXX (1964): 190–193.
- "A Modified Approach to Cardiomyotomy in Achalasia," *M. E. Med. J.*, II (1965).

Haddad, Fuad S.

- "X-Ray in Neurosurgical Diagnosis Ventriculography," *Annual Report of the Oriental Hospital*, VIII (1956): 31–37.
- (with J. J. Haijar) "La Ventriculographie Gazeuse dans la Localization des Tumeurs Intracraniennes," *Revue Médicale du Moyen Orient*, XIII (1956): 77–78.
- "Hydatid Disease of the Brain, Some Considerations of Its Recurrence," *Archives Internationales de la Hydatidosis*, XVI (1957): 445–447.
- "Anterior Sacral Meningocele, Report of Two Cases and Review of the Literature," *Canadian Journal of Surgery*, I (1958): 230–242.
- (with P. Gloor and C. Tsai) "An Assessment of the Value of Sleep-Electroencephalography for Diagnosis of Temporal Lobe Epilepsy," *Electroencephalography and Clinical Neurophysiology*, X (1958): 633–648.
- (with R. Murray) "Hydatid Disease of the Spine," *Journal of Bone and Joint Surgery*, XLI-B (1959): 499–506.
- "Quelques Remarques sur les Tumeurs Intracraniennes au Liban," *Revue Médicale du Moyen Orient*, XVI (1959): 253–259.
- (with Ph. Issa) "Pronostic Fonctionnel dans les Cas de Compression Médullaire Lente par Tumeurs Traitées Chirugicalement ou par Radiothérapie," *Revue Médicale du Moyen Orient*, XVI (1959): 78–82.
- (with W. Sinno) "A Propos d'une Compression Chiasmétique au Cours de la Grossesse," *Revue Médicale du Moyen Orient*, XVII (1960): 215–217.
- (with A. Abou Haidar) "Arfonad as an Adjunct in Surgical Treatment of Brain Tumour," *Proceedings of the 10th Middle East Medical Assembly* (1960): 143–150.
- "Preliminary Statistical Study of 209 Brain Tumors Operated upon in Lebanon," *Proceedings of the 10th Middle East Medical Assembly* (1960): 508–529.
- "Brain Tumours in the Middle East," *Annual Report of the Oriental Hospital*, XV (1962): 16–27.
- "Chronic Subdural Hematoma—A Review of 58 Cases," *Annual Report of the Oriental Hospital*, XVI (1963): 1213–1216, 1233–1235. Reprinted in *Acta Med. Iran.*, VII (1964): 19–25.
- (with C. N. Shealy and Marjorie Lewis) "Posterior Scalloping of Vertebral Bodies in Uncontrolled Hydrocephalus," *J. Neurosurg. Psychiat.*, XXVII (1964): 567–573.
- (with S. E. Kerr and G. A. Kfoury) "A Comparison of the Polyphosphoinositide in Human and Ox Brain," *Biochimica et Biophysica Acta*, LXXXIV (1964): 461–463.

Hovnanian, Auguste P.

- "The Making of a Surgeon," *Leb. Med. J.*, IV (1951): 308–311.
- "A Simple Technique for Removal of Fine Interrupted Skin Sutures," *Plast. Reconstr. Surg.*, VIII (1951): 407–408.

- "Radical Ilio-Inguinnal Node Dissection," *Ann. Surg.*, CXXXV (1952): 520–527.
- "Myxoma of the Maxilla," *Oral Surg.*, VI (1953): 927–936.
- (with I. K. Dagher) "Intrabiliary Rupture of Hydatid Cyst of the Liver," *Ann. Surg.*, CXLI (1955): 263–267.
- (with H. S. Halebian) "A Technique of Extension of Groin Incisions into the Pelvis, as Used in Regional Vascular Surgery," *J. Int. Colt. Surg.*, XXIII (1955): 93–97.
- "A Simple Technique of Skin Retraction in Selected Flap Dissections," *J. Int. Coll. Surg.*, XXIV (1955): 476–478.
- "Latissimus Dorsi Transplantation for Loss of Flexion or Extension at the Elbow: a Preliminary Report on Technic," *Ann. Surg.*, CXLIII (April 1956): 493–499.

Jidejian, Yervant D.

- *Complete Documentation on Hydatid Cyst* (a color motion picture, 1965).
- (with W. Bickers) "Transplantation of the Ureters into the Rectosigmoid," *Surg. Gynec. Obstet.*, LXXXV (1947): 30–34.
- "Transplantation of the Ureters into the Rectosigmoid," *Leb. Med. J.*, III (1950): 1–6.
- "The Prostate Gland and Its Surgery," *Leb. Med. J.*, IV (1951): 232–239.
- "Hydatid Disease," *Leb. Med. J.*, IV (1952): 59–63.
- (with J.J. McDonald) "Present Trends in Gastro-Duodenal Surgery," *Leb. Med. J.*, V (1952): 163–176.
- "Hydatid Disease," *Surgery*, XXXIV (1953): 155–167.
- "Cardiac Arrest during Surgery with Report of Four Cases," *Leb. Med. J.*, VIII (1954): 335–342.
- "Collective Review of Hydatid Disease," *J. Int. Coll. Surg.*, XXVIII (1957): 125–133.

Mcdonald, Joseph J., dean of the School of Medicine, 1953–1967; dean of the Faculties of Medical Sciences, 1953–1961; professor of surgery

- (with J. C. Chusid) *Correlative Neuroanatomy and Functional Neurology*, 12th ed. (Los Altos, California: Lange Medical Publications, 1964).
- (with J. L. Wilson) *Handbook of Surgery* (Los Altos, California: Lange Medical Publications, 1960). Second ed. 1964.
- *Development of the Nervous System*: a 16 mm, silent, black-and-white medical teaching film (1939).
- *Development of the Face and Mouth*: a 16 mm, silent, black-and-white medical teaching film (1940).
- *Development of the Gastro-Intestinal Tract*, and accompanying film on *Anomalies of the Gastro-Intestinal Tract*, a 16 mm, silent, color medical teaching film (1946); sound version (1953).

- (with B. J. Anson and L. A. Beaton) "The Origin of the Pectoralis Minor," *J. Anat.* (Lond.), LXXII (1938): 628–630.
- (with L. W. Sauer) "A Midsummer Respiratory Infection in an Aseptically Conducted Adoption Nursery," *J. Pediat.*, XIV (1939): 304–306.
- (with B. J. Anson) "Variations in the Origin of Arteries Derived from the Aortic Arch," *Amer. J. Phys. Anthrop.*, XXVII (1940): 91–107.
- (with J. P. Webster) "Early Covering of Extensive Traumatic Deformities of the Hand and Foot," *Plast. Reconstr. Surg.*, I (1946): 49–57.
- (with E. F. Cadman and J. Scudder) "The Importance of Whole Blood Transfusions in the Management of Severe Burns," *Ann. Surg.*, CXXIV (1946): 332–353.
- (with A. Z. Nsouli) "Early Postoperative Ambulation," *Rev. Méd. Liban.*, II (1949): 17–19.
- (with V. Bakamjian) "A Comparative Study of Surgical Suture Material," *Leb. Med. J.*, I (July 1950).
- "Acute Hemolytic Streptococcal Gangrene," *Leb. Med. J.*, I (November 1950).
- (with O. Friedlieb) "Ectopia Covdis (a Case Report)," *Surgery*, XXVIII (1950): 864–866.
- (with A. O. Kouyoumdjian) "Association of Congenital Adrenal Neuroblastoma with Multiple Anomalies, Including an Unusual Oropharyngeal Cavity (Imperforate Buccopharyngeal Membrane)," *Cancer* (NY), IV (1951): 784–788.
- (with Y. D. Jidejian) "Present Trends in Gastro-Duodenal Surgery," *Leb. Med. J.*, III (1952): 163–176.
- (with B. S. Azoury) "Interscapulothoracic Amputation for Osteochondroma of the Head of the Humerus," *Leb. Med. J.*, III (1952): 184–191.
- (with J. J. Haagensen and A. P. Stout) "Metastases from Mammary Carcinoma to the Supraclavicular and Internal Mammary Lymph Nodes," *Surgery*, XXXIV (1953): 521–542.
- (with D. K. McAfee and B. J. Anson) "Variation in the Point of Bifurcation of the Common Carotid Artery," *Quart. Bull. Northw. Univ. Med. Sch.*, XXVII (1953): 226–229.
- (with R. Lattes and E. Sproul) "Non-Chromoffin Paraganglioma of Carotid Body and Orbit (Case Report)," *Ann. Surg.*, CXXXIX (1954): 382–384.
- (with G. F. Crikelair) "Nasopharyngeal Chordorma, Plastic and Reconstructive," *Surgery*, XVI (1955): 138–144.
- (with I. K. Dagher) "Ankylosis of the Temporomandibular Joint," *Oral Surg.*, X (1957): 1145–1155.
- "The American University of Beirut School of Medicine," *J. Med. Educ.*, XXXIII (1958): 761–770.
- (with J. P. Webster) "Plastic Reconstruction in Cancer Surgery of the Head and Neck," in G. T. Pack and I. M. Ariel, eds., *Tumors of the Head and Neck* (New York: P. B. Hoeber Inc., 1959), 363–389.
- (with J. L. Wilson) "Medical Education in the Arab Middle East," *J. Med. Educ.*, XXXVI (1961): 1177–1199.

Mishalany, Henry G.

- (with F. Haddad) "Ureterocele in Children and Adults," *A. R. Orient Hosp.*, XII (1959): 59.
- (with F. Haddad) "Chryptorchidism and its Treatment," *A. R. Orient Hosp.*, XII (1959): 72.
- (with I. K. Dagher) "Mechanisms of Pulmonary Hypertension in Acute Hypoxia," *Proc. Xth M.E.M.A.* (1960): 469–488.
- (with F. S. Haddad, H. Boulos, and S. I. Haddad) "Volvulus of the Intestines," *A. R. Orient Hosp.*, XIV (1961): 5–12.
- (with I. K. Dagher and F. Simeone) "Mechanisms of Pulmonary Hypertension in Acute Hypoxia," *J. Thorac. Cardiovase. Surg.*, XLII (1961): 743–754.
- "Fecal Fistulas of the Scrotum in Children, Secondary to Ruptured Appendicitis," *Ann. Surg.*, CLVII (1963): 473–475.
- (with J. Bitar, B. Brandstater, S. Hajj, and M. S. Slim) "Congenital Anomalies: Etiology, Diagnosis and Surgical Considerations," *M. E. Med. J.*, II (1965): 24–42.
- "Hirschsprung's Disease (Megacolon) in the Newborn Infant," *M. E. Med. Forum*, (in press).

Mnaymneh, Walid A.

- (with H. R. Dudley and L. Ghandur–Mnaymneh) "Giant Cell Tumor of Bone," *J. Bone Jt Surg.*, XLVI–A (1964): 63–75.

Nsouli, Afif Z.

- (with J. J. McDonald) "Early Postoperative Ambulation," *Rev. Méd. Liban.*, II (1949): 17–19.
- "Low Back Pain," *Leb. Med. J.*, XV (1962): 38–44.

Obeid, Sami J.

- (with C. O. Haagensen) "Biopsy of the Apex of the Axilla in Carcinoma of the Breast," *Ann. Surg.*, CLIX (1959): 149–161.
- "The Management of a Lump in the Breast," *Leb. Med. J.*, XIV (1961): 308–313.

Slim, Michel

- "Thoracic Emergencies in the Newborn Period. A Look at the Importance and Results of Treatment of Some of the Underlying Disorders," *Leb. Med. J.*, XVI (1963): 149–161.

- (with H. D. Yacoubian, J. L.Wison, G. A.Rubeiz, and L. Ghandour- Mnaymmneh) "Successful Bilateral Reimplantation of the Canine Lungs," *Surg.* LV (1964): 676–683. [Refer to my comment on this research under Dr. H. D. Yacoubian.]
- (with J. Bitar and H. Idriss) "Hypertrophy of the Pyloric Mucosa. A Rare Cause of Congenital Pyloric Obstruction," *Amer. J. Dis Clid*, CVII (1964): 636–639.
- (with R. E. Melhem) "Congenital Pulmonary Air Cysts—Successful Segmental Resection in 50-Day-Old Infant," *Arch. Surg.*, LXXXVIII (1964): 826–923.
- (with S. S. Najjar and I. Kiblawi) "Cushing's Syndrome due to Bilateral Adrenal Hypertrophy in Childhood. Report of a Case and Review of the Literature," *Leb. Med. J.*, XVII (1964): 311–326.
- (with J. Bitar, B. Brandstater, S.Hajj, and H. G.Mishalani) "Congenital Anomalies: Etiology, Diagnosis, and Surgical Considerations," *M. E. Med. J.*, II (1965): 24–42.
- (with S. Firzliand and R. E. Melhem) "Staphylococcic Pneumonia in Infants under the Age of Six Months," *Dis Chest.*, XLV (1965): 6–13.

Whipple, Allen O.

- "The Differential Diagnosis of the Splenophathies in Relation to Their Therapy," *J. Palest. Arab Med. Ass.*, II (1947): 83.

Wilson, John L.; acting dean of the School of Medicine, 1963–1964; dean of the Faculties of Medical Sciences, 1966–); professor of surgery

- (with J. J. McDonald) *Handbook of Surgery* (Los Atlos, California: Lange Medical Publications, 1960). Second ed. (1963).
- "Survey of Results of Treatment of Gastric Cancer in San Francisco," *Calif. Med.*, CLXXIII (1950): 148.
- "Stenosing Peptic Esophagitis, with a Report of the Results of Treatment in 22 Cases," *Laryngoscope*, LXI (1951): 423–447.
- (with L. G. Brizzolara) "Carcinoma of the Tongue," *Ann. Surg.*, CXXXVI (1952): 964–970.
- (with J. Yee and P. R. Westdahl) "Gangrene of the Forearm and Hand following Use of Radial Artery for Intra-Arterial Transfusion; A Case Report," *Ann. Surg.*, CXXXVI (1952): 1019–1023.
- (with E. Barsamian) "Burns and Their Management," *Leb. Med. J.*, VII (1954): 343–359.
- (with R. A. Tabbara) "The Surgical Treatment of Heart Disease," *Leb. Med. J.*, IX (1956): 131–180.
- (with J. Srouji and R. E. Melhim) "Hydatid Cyst of the Lung with Bronchographic Evaluation of Treatment by Internal Suture of the Pericyst," *J. Thorac. Surg.*, XXXV (1958): 779–794.

- "Health and History in the Middle East," *New Engl. J. Med.*, CCLX (1959): 751–757, 811–814.
- (with C. M. Herrod, G. L. Searle, T. V. Feichtmeir, W. A. Reilly, and M. Wallner) "The Absorption of Blood from the Pleural Space," *Surgery*, XLVIII (1960): 766–774.
- "A Scapular Attachment for the Finochietto Rib Spreader," *Dis. Chest*, XXXVIII (1960): 165–166.
- (with J. M. Erskine and M. Thoshinsky) "Rupture of Aortic Homografts into the Small Intestine," *Ann. Surg.*, CLII (1960): 991–997.
- (with R. G. Stanek and W. L. Rogers) "Spontaneous Pneumothorax: A Review of 71 Cases," *Dis. Chest*, XL (1961): 391–396.
- (with J. J. McDonald) "Medical Education in the Arab Middle East," *J. Med. Educ.*, XXXVI (1961): 1171–1191.
- (with A. S. Geha) "Present Status of Portacaval Shunt in Cirrhosis," *M. E. Med. J.*, I (1962): 57–66.
- (with S. S. Saleh, H. D. Yacoubian, I. K. Dagher, and L. Ghandur-Mnaymneh) "The Absorption of Blood from the Pericardium," *J. Thorac. Cardiovasc. Surg.*, XLIV (1962) 785–792, 810–812. [**Nassar comment:** According to the authors, hemopericardium secondary to trauma or cardiac surgery clinically has been proven that it can be absorbed and may not require removal unless cardiac tamponade is present. The purpose of this research was to study how whole blood absorption from the pericardium occurs; a process not studied previously, whereas electrolytes and dyes are readily removed by the plexuses of pericardial lymphatics at the base of the pericardium and by subepicardial lymphatics.]
- (coauthor) "Gastro-Intestinal Tract and Liver," in H. Brainerd, S. Margen, and M. J. Chatton, eds., *Current Diagnosis and Treatment*, 3rd ed. (Los Altos, California: Lange Medical Publications, 1964), 306–374.
- "Diseases of the Breast," in H. Brainerd, S. Margen, and M. J. Chatton, eds., *Current Diagnosis and Treatment*, 3rd ed. (Los Altos, California: Lange Medical Publications, 1964), 375–381.
- (coauthor) "Diseases due to Physical Agents," in H. Brainerd, S. Margen, and M. J. Chatton, eds., *Current Diagnosis and Treatment*, 3rd ed. (Los Altos, California: Lange Medical Publications, 1964), 382–794.
- (with M. S. Slim, H. D. Yacoubian, G. A. Rubeiz, and L. Ghandur-Mnaymneh) "Successful Bilateral Reimplantation of the Canine Lungs," *Surgery*, LV (1964): 676–683.

Yacoubian, Hagop D.

- (with T. Dajani) "Preliminary Report on a New Method of Surgical Management of Hydatid Cysts of the Lung," *Ann. Surg.*, CLVII (1963): 618–624.
- (with M. S. Slim, J. L. Wilson, G. A. Rubeiz, and L. Ghandur-Mnaymneh) "Successful Bilateral Reimplantation of the Canine Lungs," *Surgery*, LV (1964): 676–683. [**Nassar**

comment: Review of this experimental research work showed that bilateral lung reimplantation in the dog is a real possibility, with little effect on lung function after denervation, and except for mild increased veno arterial admixture and reduced compliance, which were reversible with passage of time (months) after surgery. It may open an avenue for future research on lung transplantation in end-stage obstructive lung disease.]

- (with J. L. Wilson, S. S. Saleh, I. K. Saleh, I. K. Dagher, and L. Ghandur-Mnaymneh) "The Absorption of Blood from the Pericardium," *J. Thorac. Cardiovasc. Surg.*, XLIV (1962): 785–792, 810–812.

SECTION 1: A Prelude—My Personal Journey

My Research Experience as It Evolved in the American University School of Arts and Sciences; Faculty of Medicine of American University of Beirut; Beirut, Lebanon

A Prelude to My Journey into Medical Research

Following my graduation with the high school diploma from the international college in 1951 (which was part of the American University of Beirut, AUB, then), I enrolled in the freshman class of the School of Arts and Sciences of AUB on a reduced schedule of courses because I was not really prepared for the free academic environment of the university. I completed the remaining two freshman courses at the summer session. I did well in all and was promoted to the sophomore class, which also was extended to the summer session of that year for an extensive course in physical chemistry. I found the sophomore class very appealing and did well in the sciences, and equally well in the humanities general education course titled, Biennial Lecture Series of Western Civilization.

One of the English teachers, Professor Newman, was very much interested in the novel *Moby Dick* by Herman Melville. He required the students to read the novel and write a research term paper on any character of the novel, but in particular on Captain Ahab.

The novel clearly plays out a tragic drama; Captain Ahab, a tragic hero, pursuing a white whale for the kill, a personal vendetta. The shipmates were in awe and fear of the one-legged captain. The whale, in a previous encounter with Ahab, bit one leg off, but the captain was able to extract a tooth from the whale, which was transplanted for the missing leg of the captain. The whale hunt sea excursion was centered on the pursuit of Moby Dick by the reclusive, obsessed, vengeful Captain Ahab.

Ishmael recounts how Moby Dick and Ahab became one in the final encounter, due to a mishap. Ahab's leg became entangled by the harpoon rope, which yanked him from the ship's deck out to sea, unto his nemesis, Moby Dick. Both disappeared into the depths of the sea.

I likened those events to the ancient mariner in Samuel Taylor Coleridge's epic poem saga, *The Rhyme of the Ancient Mariner*, where he survived, like Ishmael, to tell the story of the cursed ship and its encounter with the albatross, to the company of a wedding party ashore. He was an uninvited guest, whose listeners stared at him with disbelief as if he were a man coming from the throes of death.

It is an unexplainable mystery of creation where, according to Genesis, God created good and evil and gave man free choice. Man's disobedience resulted in original, cursed sin, where man brought pain, suffering, and death, even though God had cautioned and warned Adam and Eve of the consequences if they swayed from his counsel.

However, the ancient mariner, unlike Ahab, realized the mistake of killing the albatross that brought severe distress and death. The ship's crew considered the bird a good omen to start. Its death brought the ship to a standstill with no wind or drinking water. The ancient mariner recalled the commandment "thou shalt not kill." He repented, and he began to admire the slimy creatures surrounding the motionless ship as God's creation, and the dead crew on the parched deck without a drop of water to drink, also, as part of God's creation. Man has to conquer the evil within himself, with the free choice given to him by the Creator.

Then, the ancient mariner continued: Without warning the ship came to life, and the sails started flapping in response to a change in the weather and blowing wind, guiding the ship to safe harbor.

After submitting my paper, several anxious days passed before Professor Newman announced, in front of the class of ninety students, that there is a student amongst you (Munir Nassar) who may one day make his mark and excel in life. His term paper on Moby Dick is A+, the highest grade in the class.

In the junior class, I matriculated in the sciences and was admitted to the senior class as a conjoint as also first-year medicine in 1954–1955 of the Faculty of Medicine of AUB. During the summer vacation of that year (1955), I reviewed the physiology and biochemistry units and was quizzed verbally on those subjects by Drs. Badeer and Kerr, and scored highly with them. They concluded by asking me my opinion about what is important in maintaining normal health and in disease. I replied, "The delivery of the important nutritional elements that sustain normal cell function with provision of normal oxygenation of the organs of the human being."

Continuation: My Journey in Medical Research

In 1956–1957, I was approached by Dr. Samir Azzam, a medical residency staff member at AUB, with the news that Drs. André Cournand and Dickinson W. Richards of Columbia University in New York were awarded the Nobel Prize in medicine or physiology. Their work was a first in utilizing the method of right heart catheterization in the study of heart disease. My first reaction to Dr. Azzam, though congratulatory, was that the first doctor to introduce right heart catheterization as a method for physiological investigation was a German, Dr.

Werner Frossmann. The following day I learned that Dr. Frossmann was also included among the awardees. Several years later, Dr. Richards became my mentor.

During my third year of medicine in the Medical School (now Faculty of Medicine) of the AUB, I became aware of the many contributions of Dr. Sami I. Haddad.

I was introduced to Ibn Nafis by one of our teachers during my third year of medical schooling, and I became fascinated with, and an admirer of Dr. Sami I. Haddad for his research on Ibn Nafis, which was accomplished in 1936, when Dr. Haddad was a member of the American University Senate, and associate professor of surgery and fellow of the American College of Surgeons. Later on in his career, he became professor of surgery and chairman of the Department of Surgery, and dean, and chief of staff at the AUB School of Medicine (now Faculty of Medicine) and University Hospital.

I mentioned Dr. Sami I. Haddad because, during my fellowship at Columbia University College of Physicians and Surgeons (1963–1965), I was approached by Drs. Dickinson W. Richards (my mentor), André Cournand, and Alfred P. Fishman to verify and explain the Arabic text that was translated into English of the *Commentary of Ibn Nafis*, on the *Canon* of Ibn Sina, dealing with the discovery of the pulmonary circulation. I found out after researching the subject that the translated English text was accurate, according to the paper of Dr. Sami I. Haddad. The translated Arabic to English text was published in their book *Circulation of the Blood; Men and Ideas*. Subsequently, I wrote a brief paper on Ibn Nafis, which was published in the *Journal of the Royal Society of Medicine* and a lengthy manuscript submitted to the Rochester Academy of Medicine in 2001.

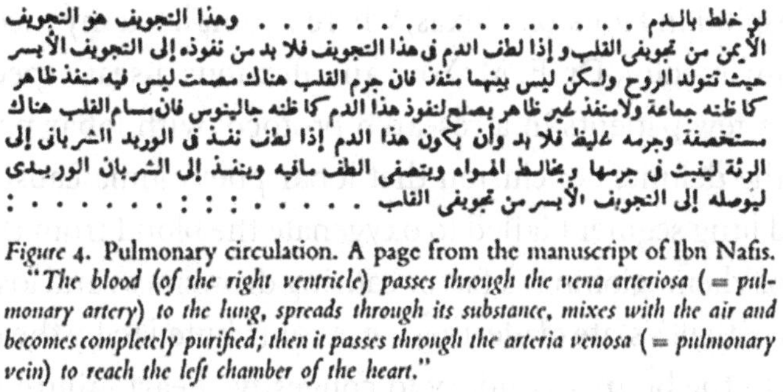
لو خلط بالدم . . . . وهذا التجويف هو التجويف
الأيمن من تجويفى القلب وإذا لطف الدم فى هذا التجويف فلا بد من نفوذه إلى التجويف الأيسر
حيث تتولد الروح ولكن ليس بينهما منفذ فان جرم القلب هناك مصمت ليس فيه منفذ ظاهر
كما ظنه جماعة ولا منفذ غير ظاهر يصلح لنفوذ هذا الدم كما ظنه جالينوس فان مسام القلب هناك
مستحصفة وجرمه غليظ فلا بد وأن يكون هذا الدم إذا لطف نفذ فى الوريد الشريانى إلى
الرئة لينبث فى جرمها ويخالط الهواء ويتصفى ألطف مائيه وينفذ إلى الشريان الوريدى
ليوصله إلى التجويف الأيسر من تجويفى القلب . . . . . . : : : . . . . :

Figure 4. Pulmonary circulation. A page from the manuscript of Ibn Nafis.
"The blood (of the right ventricle) passes through the vena arteriosa (= pulmonary artery) to the lung, spreads through its substance, mixes with the air and becomes completely purified; then it passes through the arteria venosa (= pulmonary vein) to reach the left chamber of the heart."

[15]

The above is the Arabic text of Ibn Nafis commentary and English translation. Alfred P. Fisman and Dickinson W. Richards, eds., *Circulation of the Blood: Men and Ideas* (Oxford University Press, New York, 1964), ch. 1, "Air and Blood," Andre Cournand.

I am getting ahead of myself here. These papers on Ibn Nafis will be discussed later during the time of my research in the United States.

During my fourth year in medicine at AUB, I helped on a paper involving fifteen cases of polycystic kidney disease in Lebanon authored by Drs. Fuad Bashour and Samir Azzam. The paper was not published. However, its application to clinical medicine was that the diagnosis of polycystic kidneys can be made when palpable upper quadrant masses of the abdomen are noted on exam associated with elevated blood pressure and compromised renal function.

During my medical internship, we desensitized a patient from his allergy to penicillin under the supervision of Dr. Fuad Farah. After completion of a Rockefeller Foundation scholarship at Barne's Hospital, Dr. Farah later on developed the first immunological research center at the Faculty of Medicine of AUB, a first in Lebanon—another milestone example in the development of research due to the vision and initiative of Dr. Farah.

As senior medical resident, I was given the task of a lecturer to third- and fourth-year medical students on heart failure, part of their biennial lecture series. In addition to giving the classical pathophysiologic explanation of heart failure leading to lung congestion/edema, hepatomegaly with peripheral pitting edema of the ankles, I introduced the concept of altered metabolic function of contractile cardiac muscle (actin and myosin) (the concept of free energy from ATP degraded to ADP and its acceptance of phosphate from phosphocreatine). [R. J. Bing, "The Metabolism of the Heart," *The Harvey Lectures 1954* (New York Academic Press, 1956.)]

The pathologist at the AUB Hospital, Dr. L. Ghandour, asked me to discuss a patient from the hospital records at the clinical pathological conference, a seventy-eight-year-old white male patient who entered the hospital with unconsciousness and was found to have lobar pneumonia and congestive heart failure.

At the Methodist Hospital in Houston, Texas, where I completed my medical residency, I had worked closely with my mentor, Dr. E. M. Yow, an infectious disease specialist who in a small way helped work up a few patients in a research protocol with lobar pneumonia. The study was published with the definite conclusion that lobar pneumonia causes shunting of blood, whereby the perfused lung segment failed to oxygenate the blood from the pulmonary artery, and the unsaturated oxyhemoglobin is a factor causing drowsiness and loss of consciousness. It was obvious that this patient's state of alertness was contributed to by the pneumonia infection with poor perfusion to the brain secondary to congestive heart failure [J. K. Alexander and coworkers, "Studies on Pulmonary Blood Flow in Pneumococcal Pneumonia," *Cardio Vasc. Research Bull.* 1 (1963): 86]. **Nassar comment:** I introduced the myocardial infarction markers creatine phosphokinase (CPK) and lactic dehydrogenase (LDH) to the professors attending my clinical pathological conference. Recent advances expound troponin 1 and troponin T laboratory tests as more accurate markers to detect acute myocardial infarction. Those tests were not known then. Be that as it may, the patient's congestive heart failure could be on the basis of infarction. Refer to my Epilogue discussion of congestive heart failure prompted by Dr. G. Fawaz's synthesis of phosphocreatine.

So far I have tried to establish that scholarly clinical research was active and continuing at AUB but was not popularized in contradistinction to the emphasis on the importance of medical teaching and educating budding physicians. To wit, and to buttress my point for the development of medical research, I cite the following examples to show the progress of research.

George Fawaz, MD, PhD, chairman and professor of pharmacology at AUB (1949–1984), published original work on the synthesis of phosphocreatine, among more than ninety-two publications of medical and educational significance. Also, he developed an antimalarial drug, Lapinone, for the treatment of plasmodium vivax malaria. In 1967, I discussed with Professor Fawaz the possibility of doing research on urokinase. However, no funds were available to carry on such research. **Nassar comment:** Urokinase is a naturally occurring substance produced by the renal cell parenchyma and excreted in the urine. It can be extracted from the urine and purified, and after decontamination maybe used intravenously as a clot disintegrator of fibrin clot in patients with acute coronary thrombosis infarction to reestablish coronary blood flow in the occluded artery.

Urokinase
$\downarrow$
a-Plasminogen---------> Plasmin

Plasmin
$\downarrow$
b-Fibrinogen … … … > Fibrin clot (busted)

Dr. Fawaz was a distinguished scholar and one of the pillars of AUB and its medical education and research.

The Faculty of Medicine was indeed fortunate during that period of time to have Dean Joseph J. McDonald, MD, Dr. Med. Sc., formerly, professor of surgery at Columbia College of Physicians and Surgeons, a leader whose vision enriched the Faculty of Medicine.

Dr. McDonald was assisted by Dr. John L. Wilson (Harvard), a cardiothoracic surgeon who, with local faculty physicians Ibrahim Dagher (Mayo Clinic and Cleveland Clinic), George A. Rubeiz (Harvard), Riad Tabbara (Harvard), and others, developed cardiac surgery and the cardiology departments at the hospital.

The risk factors of heart disease are smoking, weight, elevated lipids (cholesterol), hypertension, diabetes mellitus, and history of heart disease. Any one of these risk factors can be found between the ages of 12–19 and thereafter. This is according to the American Heart Association and the Centers for Disease Control in the United States. Also, it is to be noted that, though mortality from heart disease has been reduced, these risk factors remain high. The census according to the American Heart Association is that mortality from heart disease and stroke occur daily with these figures: 2,200 and 360 respectively.

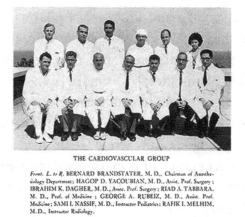

THE CARDIOVASCULAR GROUP

Front. L. to R. BERNARD BRANDSTATER, M. D., Chairman of Anesthesiology Department; HAGOP D. YACOUBIAN, M. D., Asist. Prof. Surgery; IBRAHIM K. DAGHER, M. D., Assoc. Prof. Surgery; RIAD A. TABBARA, M. D., Prof. of Medicine; GEORGE A. RUBEIZ, M. D., Asist. Prof. Medicine; SAMI I. NASSIF, M. D., Instructor Pediatrics; RAFIK I. MELHIM, M. D., Instructor Radiology.

Back. L. to R. JOHN L. WILSON, M.D., Prof. Surgery; JOSEPH HOBEIKA, Lab.Technician; SUHAYL SALEH, M.D., Research Fellow; TAHER DAJANI, M. D., Resident Surgery; MUNIR NASSAR, M. D., Research Fellow; ASDGHIG LERCHIGIAN, Research Assistant.

The above is a photo of members of the cardiac surgery team.

Dr. Ibrahim Dagher is accredited with the development of a first in the Middle East: a rotator disc oxygenator for the heart-lung machine that was used routinely in open-heart surgery. He was assisted in its development by Dr. F. J. Dagher. He reported on open cardiac repair on ten cases of Tetralogy of Fallot, again a first in Lebanon and the Middle East.

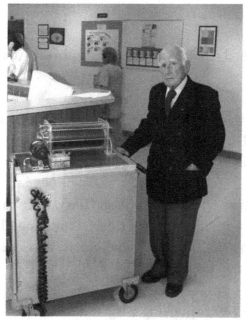

■ Dr. Ibrahim Dagher standing next to the cardiopulmonary bypass machine he designed in 1958.

The above is a photo of the membrane oxygenator for heart-lung machine.
[*AUBMC News*, vol. 11, no. 3 (June 2007).

The Cardiovascular Program became a reality and was supported by grants from the National Institute of Health, Bethesda, Maryland; the American Heart Association; and others. Among its goals: to gather basic data and to foster clinical and laboratory research (1961–1962).

One of the main research projects was The Study of Rheumatic Heart Disease in Lebanon. I was a research fellow assisting Drs. J. L. Wilson and G. A. Rubeiz in the cardiopulmonary catheterization laboratory of AUH.

I developed an IBM protocol on cards for this study. However, Dr. Wilson elected to report on the surgical treatment of mitral stenosis using the surgical method (mitral commissurotomy) on each of 329 patients out of a total of 441 patients studied medically. The first cardiac surgery, i.e., mitral commissurotomy, was in 1954; truly a first open-heart surgery in Lebanon and the Middle East.

Table 1. Number of Operations per Year	
Year	Number of Operations
1954	1
1955	4
1956	5
1957	11
1958	10
1959	32
1960	29
1961	53
1962	52
1963	62
1964	62
1965	8
TOTAL	329 (Of this total, 157 patients had mitral valve stenosis without associated other forms of cardiac valve disorder.)

Table 2. Preoperative Cardiac Classification, according to the New York Heart Association		
Class	Number	Percent
II	51	32
III	88	56
IV	18	12
Total	157	100%

Table 3. Frequency of Post-Operative Atrial Fibrillation in Ninety-Four Patients Studied with Preoperative Normal Sinus Rhythm.

Post-operative atrial fibrillation -------------------- 26 or 28%

Normal sinus rhythm ----------------------------- 68 or 72%

Table 4. Major Preoperative Complications

Peripheral embolization---------------------------- 13 or 8%

Absence of peripheral embolization--------------- 144 or 92%

--------------------Total---------------------------- 157 or 100%

Table 5. Surgical Approach

Left anterior thoracotomy------------------------- 144 or 92%

Median sternotomy ------------------------------- 6 or 4%

Bilateral thoracotomy ---------------------------- 4 or 2%

Right thoracotomy ------------------------------- 3 or 2%

--------------------Total---------------------------- 157 or 100%

Table 6. Diagnosis of Mitral Valve Lesion at Surgery

Pure mitral stenosis ------------------------------ 115 or 73%

Major mitral stenosis, minor insufficiency--------- 39 or 25%

Significant mitral insufficiency, minor stenosis --- 3 or 25%

Table 7. Postoperative Complications

Atelectasis and/or pneumonia --------------------- 34

Atrial fibrillation --------------------------------- 26

Congestive heart failure---------------------------- 7

Infection --------------------------------------- 4

Peripheral embolization---------------------------- 3

Hemorrhage ------------------------------------- 2

This clinical surgical study demonstrates the actuality that reporting on data gives an impetus for the continuation of research outcomes.

Comments on Certain References in Chapter 3

Various Faculty Members' Published Papers in Cardiology with Which I Was Involved

The clinical significance of the post-extra systolic T wave changes that follow a normally conducted PQRST beat was found to correlate with heart disease. Coronary artery disease being most frequent heart disease suggested that such T wave phenomenon may be used as a predictor of coronary artery disease even in asymptomatic patients.

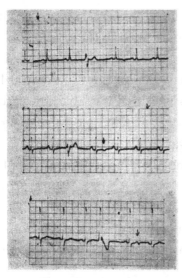

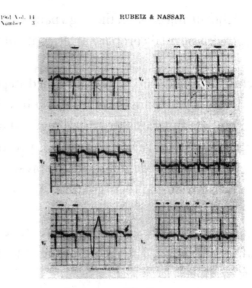

Fig. 1

There is complete reversal in the T of the normally conducted beat that follows **the ventricular** premature systole in lead V5 and lead II. The patient is fifty-five years old with arteriosclerotic heart disease.

Fig. 2

The precordial leads V1 - V6) on a fifty-six year old man with anterior myocardial infarction. Note reversal of T in lead V3, in the normally conducted beat that follows a ventricular premature systole.

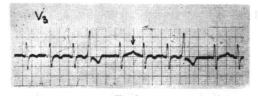

Fig. 3

Lead V3 showing a reversion to positive of an already negative T wave, in the normally conducted beat that follows a ventricular premature systole. The patient, fourteen years old, had acute glomerulonephritis and renal failure.

THE SIGNIFICANCE OF THE POST-EXTRA-SYSTOLIC The Lebanese Medical Journal

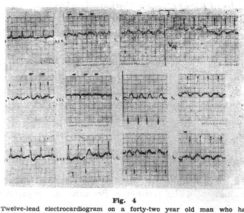

Fig. 4

Twelve-lead electrocardiogram on a forty-two year old man who had rheumatic heart disease with aortic and mitral valve affection and superimposed subacute bacterial endocarditis. Lead V4 shows a biphasic T that becomes completely negative in the normal beat that follows a ventricular premature systole.

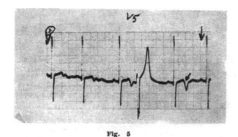

Fig. 5

V5 on a seventy year old man with arteriosclerotic heart disease exhibiting the typical post-extra-systolic T wave change.

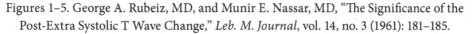

Figures 1–5. George A. Rubeiz, MD, and Munir E. Nassar, MD, "The Significance of the Post-Extra Systolic T Wave Change," *Leb. M. Journal*, vol. 14, no. 3 (1961): 181–185.

In the published paper on acute pancreatitis with electrocardiographic evidence of acute myocardial infarction, it may be possible to postulate another etiology for the observed myocardial infarction; a coronary artery embolus secondary to the atrial fibrillation as well as a small embolus to a branch of the pancreatic artery. My comment here is in no way intended to diminish the clinical observations of the authors, and the possibility of pancreatic enzyme action on the myocardium. In the emergency room, I was the doctor in charge when the patient arrived. It is interesting to note that experimental induction of pancreatitis secondary to taurocholate injection in the dog's pancreatic duct produced abnormal electrocardiographic changes with normal coronary arteries at autopsy (reference cited in the article).

The clinical application of the published paper on "The Study of the Right Atrial Pressure Pulse and Normal Sinus Rhythm" (also in mitral stenosis) is that it enables the cardiologist to differentiate functional tricuspid regurgitation from organic tricuspid valve regurgitation using superior vena cava pressure pulse recording, logarithmic phonocardiogram and the electrocardiogram to demonstrate the preservation of the A x V Y right pressure pulse curve in functional tricuspid regurgitation.

The same conclusions apply to differentiate functional mitral insufficiency from organic mitral regurgitation. The record of the left atrial venous pulse is obtained during left atrial catheterization.

RIGHT ATRIAL PRESSURE PULSE

Table 1

Results of Right Cardiac Catheterization

	S.B.	E.A.	Patient H.H.	M.Z.	S.K.
RA	m = 3	m = 3	m = 3	m = 7	m = 9
RV	86/0-3	81/0-3	113/3	100/2-7	45/9
PA	86/45 m = 70	81/34 m = 42	113/46 m = 78	100/35 m = 57	45/28 m = 34
PC	m = 30	m = 26	–	m = 35	–
CI (L./min./M.²)	1.7	2.36	2.2	2.8	2.6
PVR (dynes sec.) (cm.⁻⁵)	1360	352	–	429	–

RA, right atrium; RV, right ventricle; PA, pulmonary artery; PC, pulmonary capillary; CI, cardiac index; PVR, pulmonary vascular resistance. Pressures are expressed in mm. Hg.

Table 2

Right Atrial Pressure Pulse Components Expressed in mm. Hg

Wave	S.B.	E.A.	Patient H.H.	M.Z.	S.K.	M.N.
A	4	7	5	12	12	8
C	–	4	–	–	12	–
V	0	4	3.3	8.4	6	6

The X descent was deeper than the Y in all cases, except that in S.K. the X descent was equal to the Y descent. In four cases the C wave was not identified. Patient M.N. had only the right atrial pressure-pulse obtained at thoracotomy.

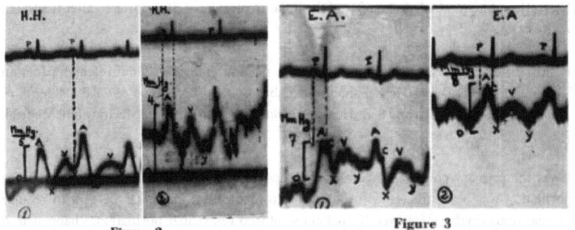

Figure 2

Figure 3

1, right atrial pressure-pulse obtained in patient H.H. at right cardiac catheterization. The X descent is well preserved. 2, the same obtained at thoracotomy.

1, right atrial pressure-pulse obtained in patient E.A. at right cardiac catheterization. The X descent is well preserved. 2, the same obtained at thoracotomy.

George A. Rubeiz, MD, Munir E. Nassar, MD, and Ibrahim K. Dagher, MD,
"Study of the Right Atrial Pressure Pulse in Functional Tricuspid Regurgitation
and Normal Sinus Rhythm," *Circulation*, XXX (August 1964).

This paper is referenced in Braunwald's *Heart Disease* textbook, 1990 edition; and in *Clinical Phonocardiography and External Pulse Recording* by Morton E. Tavel (Chicago: Year Book Publishers Inc., 1972): 50, 305.

Again, the clinical postulate that may be gleaned from the published paper, "Correlation of the Positive Two-Step Exercise Test" (reference cited in chapter 3) and the changes noted on the electrocardiogram suggested coronary artery disease secondary to severity of mitral stenosis and elevated pulmonary vascular resistance; both phenomena compromise coronary blood flow.

The causes of the positive exercise test are not so clear-cut. In active, untreated rheumatic heart disease, arteritis of the coronary arteries may occur. [D. P. White, "The Clinical Significance of Cardiac Pain," in R. L. Levy, *Diseases of the Coronary Arteries and Cardiac Pain* (New York: The Macmillan Co., 1936), 209.] However, at autopsy, Aschoff bodies were found lying close to a vessel; though not totally uncommon, panarteritis were noted in coronary arteries and other blood vessels. [P. Wood, *Diseases of the Heart and Circulation*, second revised edition (Philadelphia: J. B. Lippincott Co., 1963), 473.]

Currently, the C-reactive protein test, though a nonspecific test, denotes or is associated with inflammation. The unresolved answer to the question is whether beta hemolytic strep that initiates active rheumatic fever may be somehow also a nonspecific factor in the inflammatory coronary plaque formation. Recent evidence suggests that Lipitor and other statins have other anti-inflammatory properties besides lowering the total cholesterol and LDLs. In addition, the

C-reactive protein, which is a marker of the inflammatory process, is lowered after treatment with statins.[39]

Positive values of C-reactive protein (CRP) were a common finding in our research paper on "Rheumatic Heart Disease in Lebanon" cited above. [A positive value of CRP>0.8mg/dl as reported in L. G. Gomella and S. A. Haist, *Clinicians Pocket Reference* (McGraw Hill Medical, 2007), 53–54, 210.]

I was the primary physician involved in successfully resuscitating a patient whose atrial fibrillation was being treated with quinidine to medically convert his rhythm to regular normal sinus rhythm. However, the patient went into ventricular fibrillation. I happened to be in the medical pavilion that Saturday afternoon when the nurse alerted me, being the only doctor available, to the patient's arrest. This patient's recovery was written up and published in the *American Journal of Cardiology*. My name was excluded (reference cited in chapter 3).

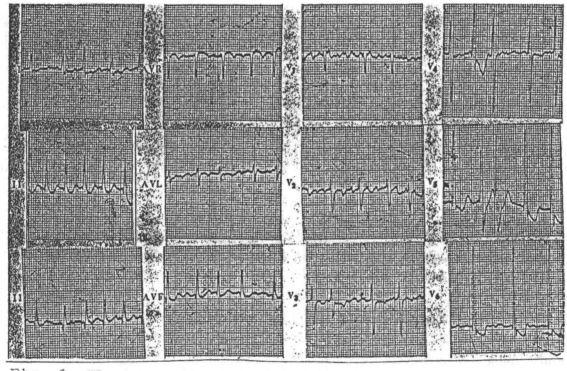

Fig. 2. Electrocardiogram on March 30, 1963.

Atrial fibrillation.

---

39 "Statins and Inflammation: an Update," *Curr Opin Cardiol*, 25(4) (July 2010): 399:405.

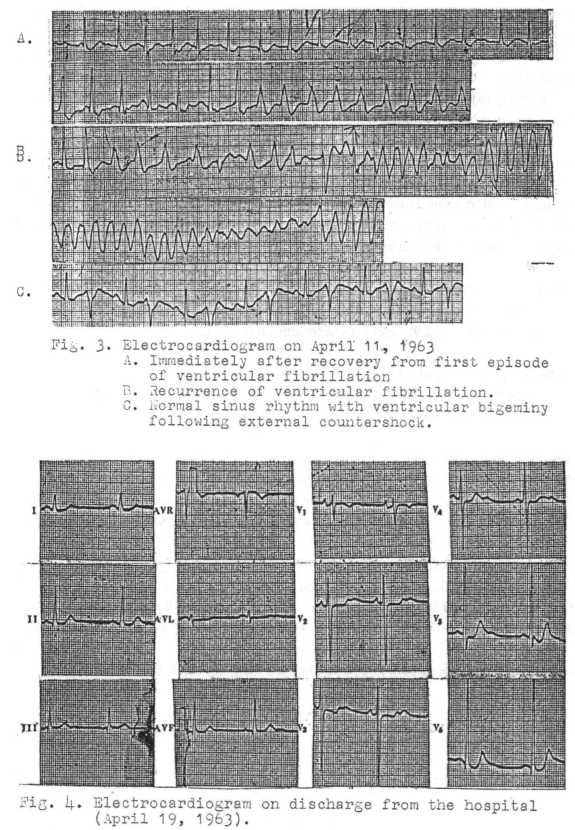

Fig. 3. Electrocardiogram on April 11, 1963
    A. Immediately after recovery from first episode of ventricular fibrillation
    B. Recurrence of ventricular fibrillation.
    C. Normal sinus rhythm with ventricular bigeminy following external countershock.

Fig. 4. Electrocardiogram on discharge from the hospital (April 19, 1963).

The treatment that was done included electric cardioversion and a rapid infusion of one liter of normal saline solution besides basic life support.

In 1967, I was fortunate to be able to work part-time at the Gulbenkian Respiratory Laboratory at the Chest Disease Hospital at Azounieh Village in Lebanon. I presented to the director of the hospital, Dr. Papken Mugrditchian, my research project to study lung function in healthy Lebanese children for the purpose of establishing prediction formulas that would be used clinically to measure lung function parameters: vital capacity, one-second expiratory volume, and maximum breathing capacity. He agreed. I was happy to have Alfred Nassar at the Computer Center of American University of Beirut, Beirut, Lebanon, who reviewed the analysis of the data, including the use of the T test and the standard deviation of the mean. Furthermore, to develop such respiratory tests was novel and a first, since none were available for Lebanese children. One hundred twenty children and adolescents were screened by history, physical exam, chest roentgenograms, and laboratory for inclusion in the study. One hundred fifteen were found healthy and were studied.

FVC for male children 10–12 years inclusive =
$$-- 1544.28 + 86.48 \text{ (age)} + 8.72 \text{ (height)} + 1651.9 \text{ (B.S.A.)}; R = 0.82 \text{ (1)}$$
$$\text{Or } --3476.49 + 122.99 \text{ (age)} + 33.12 \text{ (height)}; R = 0.77 \text{ (2)}$$

FVC for female children 10–12 years inclusive =
$$-- 3948.36 + 25.81 \text{ (age)} + 42.93 \text{ (height)} + (--122.32) \text{ (B.S.A.)}; R = 0.89 \text{ (3)}$$
$$\text{Or } 3988.81 = 32.98 \text{ (age)} + 41.67 \text{ (height)}; R = 0.88 \text{ (4)}$$

For male children: adolescents:
$$FVC = --243.57 + 62.25 \text{ (age)} + 11.30 \text{ (height)} + 2314.24 \text{ (B.S.A.)}; R = 0.923 \text{ (5)}$$
$$FEV_{1.0} = -- 3154.47 + 67.72 \text{ (age)} + 23 \text{ (height)} + 1169.54 \text{ (B.S.A.)}; R = 0.893 \text{ (6)}$$
$$MBC = --169.47 + 2.10 \text{ (age)} + 1.738 \text{ (height)} + 14.90 \text{ (B.S.A.)}; R = 0.791 \text{ (7)}$$

For female children: adolescents:
$$FVC = -- 4530.98 + 19.02 \text{ (age)} + 45.22 \text{ (height)} + 189.78 \text{ (B.S.A.)}; R = 0.870 \text{ (8)}$$
$$FEV_{1.0} = --3689.93 + 54.03 \text{ (age)} + 33.96 \text{ (height)} + 284.07 \text{ (B.S.A.)}; R = 0.886 \text{ (9)}$$
$$MBC = -- 101.49 + 3.81 \text{ (age)} + 0.813 \text{ (height)} + 8.38 \text{ (B.S.A.)}; R = 0.586 \text{ (10)}$$

(Lung volumes and capacities in mls BTPS obtained using the prediction formulas.)

TABLE I

LUNG VOLUMES AND CAPACITIES IN mls BTPS

	1200 meters altitude				Sea-level			
	Males		Females		Males		Females	
	10-12 yrs	13-15 yrs	10-12 yrs	13-15 yrs	10-12 yrs	13-15 yrs	10-12 yrs	13-15 yrs
Number of children	16	17	17	13	16	9	14	13
Age (mean)	11.4SD ± 0.5	13.9 SD ± 0.9	11.1 SD ± 0.8	13.5 SD ± 0.7	11.6 SD ± 0.5	14.1 SD ± 0.9	11.6 SD ± 0.5	13.5 SD ± 0.6
Height in cms (mean)	138SD ± 6	154 SD ± 8.9	138.7 SD ± 7.1	151 SD ± 7.7	142.2 SD ± 7.6	157 SD ± 9	145.3 SD ± 7.3	155.3 SD ± 4.8
Weight in kgms (mean)	31SD ± 3	43.7 SD ± 9	33 SD ± 6.3	41.2 SD ± 6.9	36.8 SD ± 7.1	49.4 SD ± 13.5	37.5 SD ± 10.9	49.9 SD10.6
B.S.A. in M^2	1.09SD ± 0.1	1.37 SD ± 0.2	1.13 SD ± 0.1	1.32 SD ± 0.1	1.2 SD ± 0.1	1.49 SD ± 0.2	1.2 SD ± 0.3	1.43 SD ± 0.1
$\overline{FEV}_{1.0}$	2151 SD ± 250	2868 SD ± 665	1942 SD ± 312	2528.5 SD393.2	2286 SD ± 269	3135 SD ± 699	2182 SD ± 333	2759 SD ± 361
$\overline{FVC}$	2434 SD ± 263	3252 SD ± 764	2153 SD ± 340	2762 SD ± 457	2721 SD ± 355	3579 SD868	2456 SD ± 377	3108 SD ± 445
$\overline{MBC}$ L/min	77.6 SD ± 14.6	109.5 SD ± 26	61 SD ± 23	88.5 SD ± 25	84.5 SD ± 16.1	107 SD ± 15.6	74.8 SD ± 12.8	83.3 SD ± 16
$FEV_{1.0}$ / $FVC \times 100$	88 % SD ± 3.5	88 % SD ± 6	90 % SD ± 5.1	91 % SD ± 4.5	84 % SD ± 4.7	88 % SD4.4	89 % SD ± 6	89 % SD ± 5.2

The prediction formulas for Group I at 1200 meters altitude (subdivided into females and males) and Group II at sea level (subdivided into females and males). Mounir Nassar, MD, ME, "Lung Function Norms of Lebanese Children and Adolescents," *J. Anaesth*, 2 (6) (1970): 475–491 (reference cited in chapter 3).

Continuation of a Doctor's Research Experience

Dr. Badeer, a physiologist physician, par excellence, and Dr. K. Abu Feisal reported on "The Effect of Atrial and Ventricular Tachycardia on Cardiac Oxygen Consumption," *Cir. Res.* 17 (1965): 330–335. The conclusions drawn from this study on seven mongrel dogs showed that an increase in heart rate from 130 bpm to 157 bpm during atrial tachycardia, and from 130 bpm to 158 bpm in ventricular tachycardia, increased O_2 uptake by 11.5 percent and 50 percent, respectively. Total coronary flow was greater during ventricular tachycardia from the observed measurements of atrial tachycardia at equivalent heart rates, suggesting greater energy expenditure of dogs' hearts in ventricular tachycardia.

The concept of this research activity was suggested by Dr. G. Fawaz, based on clinical discussions generated on the medical wards by Dr. Munir Nassar and Dr. K. Abu Feisal.

An earlier work, "Influence of Oxygen on Hypothermic Cardiac Standstill in the Heart-Lung Preparation," *Circ. Res.* 3 (1955): 28–31, showed that induced terminal ventricular fibrillation by hypothermia at seventeen–eighteen degrees centigrade was not influenced by increased delivery of pure O_2 (100 percent), even when alkalemia was prevented, in the heart-lung preparation of dogs.

Hence, it is quite obvious that research was well on its way. More complete bibliographical data is found in chapter 3.

Research on hyperlipidemia was generated following patients treated in the medical wards of American University Hospital, and some of the patients were presented at medical grand rounds, notably those with familial hyperlipidemia.

Dr. Avedis Khachadurian, associate professor of biochemistry and internal medicine, became interested and was actively involved in patients with hyperlipemia who were referred to the biochemistry laboratory. In 1962, Dr. Khachadurian published a literature review of the state of knowledge of essential hyperlipemia, and reported on a thirty-two-year-old male, dentist, patient with essential hyperlipemia and gout (*MEMJ*, vol. 1:13–24).

The classical clinical features can be distinguished from other forms of hyperlipemia, for example: physiologic hyperlipemia, which is found after a fatty meal with elevated neutral fats and some phospholipids in the serum resolve within eight to ten hours. There are no clinical signs here. In contrast, secondary hyperlipemia is found in association with other diseases like uncontrolled type II diabetes, von Gierke's disease, lipoid nephrosis, nephritic phase of chronic glomerulonephritis, various forms of hepatic and pancreatic disease, starvation, hypoproteinemia, and other conditions. Here, the diagnosis is of the primary disease associated with elevated secondary hyperlipemia. In most of these conditions, secondary hyperlipemia can be reversed with control of the primary disease.

Essential hypercholesterolemia is a Mendelian dominance with "incomplete" penetrance inherited disorder with markedly elevated serum cholesterol and phospholipids. Triglycerides are normal and the serum is not turbid. The patients have tender cutaneous and tendinous exanthemata and premature, early atherosclerosis. Their prognosis is poor.

At the time the paper was published, aside from therapy with a low fat diet and niacin, there were no prescribed exercises or drugs such as the statins and cholystiramine-like drugs that are available since the past decade or more, though niacin has been available for many years past.

In essential hyperlipemia, the inheritance is probably recessive type, males affected more than females, and possibly pathologically due to delayed clearance of lipids from the blood. Chemical characteristics include turbid serum, with or without fasting, and contain marked elevation of neutral fats, phospholipids, cholesterol with low to normal ratio of esters. The beta lipoproteins are increased and so are the low density lipoproteins.

Injection of heparin causes a shift in this abnormal chemistry toward normal values. The clinical features are apparent on examination: eruptive exanthemata in the skin (buttocks and extensor surfaces of extremities similar to those seen in essential hypercholesterolemia, but with a major difference in that the lesions in the latter condition do not resolve or disappear with therapy with heparin).

The dentist patient was treated with intravenous heparin for three days and then with depot heparin intramuscular. His hyperlipemia gradually resolved and the patient was discharged on a low fat diet and benemid with colchicine.

Another important published paper by Dr. Khachadurian, titled "The Inheritance of Essential Familial Hypercholesterolemia," *AM J Med*, vol. 37 (1964): 402–407, described twelve patients with high incidence of consanguinity in sibships whose inheritance pattern showed that those with marked elevations of serum cholesterol were dominant homozygous, whereas those with moderate cholesterol elevations were heterozygous.

It is of interest to note that I referred patient number 12 for inclusion in the study. I will be presenting her medical history in some detail later on.

In another paper published in the *Leb. Med. J.*, 25 (1972): 253–267, coauthored with Drs. G. Rubeiz, and Sawaya, titled "Coronary Artery Disease in the Young," one hundred patients with coronary artery disease at ages forty-five or below, the youngest were below age thirty; eighty-nine males and eleven females. Of the nine patients below age thirty, five were homozygote for familial hypercholesterolemia. Hypercholesterolemia was present in 43 percent of study group vs. 12 percent in controls. Hypertriglyceridemia was found in 32 percent vs. 16 percent in controls. Diabetes mellitus was present in 32 percent, while it was present in 2.5 percent of the controls. Hyperuricemia was present in 30 percent and in 5 percent of controls, overweight in 22 percent vs. 10 percent in controls, hypertension was present in 9 percent vs. 35 percent in controls, and smoking in 75 percent vs. 44 percent of controls.

[**Nassar comment:** Although the relationship of premature atherosclerosis was reported in the literature in relation to risk factors mentioned above, this was a special report of its kind in relation to young Lebanese adults, because it showed that in the ninety-nine subjects studied, one or more of the risk factors reported above was present.

The conclusion of that study emphasizes the importance of screening for risk factors in a population that may be susceptible to coronary atherosclerosis prior to forty-five years of age.

It is clear that, at least in 1972 and earlier in time, clinical research papers on cholesterol were underway (see references of Drs. Khayat and Khachadurian). Research at the Faculty of Medicine at AUB was already looking at premature atherosclerosis and its predisposing risk factors; also such similar studies and associated preventive measures were being contemplated by many research centers and/or medical schools across the United States.]

It is quite apparent that the revived interest in hypercholesterolemia and its relationship to coronary atherosclerosis became widespread in the United States.

In another paper, titled "The Diagnosis and Management of Hyperlipidemias, a Review Based on 12 Years' Experience in Lebanon," published by Dr. A. K. Khachadurian in the 1972 issue of the *Lebanese Medical Journal*, vol. 25: 31–54, he writes in the introduction, "The management of hyperlipidemias will be one of the major problems facing the profession in the coming years."

Again, the experience cited was based in several instances of patient referral from the hospital of the American University of Beirut (now known as the AUB Hospital Medical Center) at the time I was completing my residency in internal medicine and one year of cardiology fellowship.

During my residency-cardiology fellowship, I actively participated and gained experience assisting in open-heart surgery for pulmonary stenosis; complete repair of Tetralogy of Fallot; and repair of renal artery stenosis for the treatment of renal hypertension. But most importantly, I worked on the problem of rheumatic heart disease in Lebanon utilizing right heart catheterization and the surgical treatment of mitral stenosis headed by Drs. John Wilson, I. Dagher, and G. A. Rubeiz.

In 1967, I was appointed part-time medical-cardiology associate in the Department of Medicine of AUB.

At this juncture in my research analysis, I would like to move forward in time to the period I left the American University of Beirut and established my private medical/cardiovascular practice in Albion, New York. I was visited by a patient with familial hypercholesterolemia from Beirut, Lebanon.

Background information: The relationship of familial hypercholesterolemia (FH) to premature vascular atherosclerosis, coronary artery disease syndromes, acute myocardial infarction, hypertension, and tendon exanthemata is well documented (see references 1–4 listed below), but unknown or not discussed relating familial hypercholesterolemia to an etiologic cause of aortic valvular stenosis. The documented endothelial vascular pathologic lesion of the aorta in familial hypercholesterolemia stated in the literature is secondary to shear stress and foam cell formation streaking of cholesterol and atherosclerotic plaque formation with calcium deposits resulting in lumen narrowing and irregular endothelial surface. However, such pathologic process is not described for aortic valve endothelial surface. The normal structure of the leaflets of the aortic valve is an endothelial surface layer laid on a stratum of connective tissue and elastic fibers forming three leaflet cusps. The orifice of the left coronary artery originates from the left cusp and the right coronary from the right cusp. [**Nassar comment:** It is my opinion that hyperlipidemia may very well cause atherosclerotic plaques in the epithelial layer of the aortic cusps causing aortic valve stenosis; another uninvestigated etiology of aortic valve stenosis.]

HEART VALVES (superior view, *JAMA* 1976:235:1603)

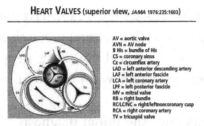

AV = aortic valve
AVN = AV node
B His = bundle of His
CS = coronary sinus
Cx = circumflex artery
LAD = left anterior descending artery
LAF = left anterior fascicle
LCA = left coronary artery
LPF = left posterior fascicle
MV = mitral valve
RB = right bundle
RC/LC/NC = right/left noncoronary cusp
RCA = right coronary artery
TV = tricuspid valve

Pocket Medicine, 4th edition (Massachusetts General Hospital Handbook of Internal Medicine, 2011).

My patient was a sixty-five-year-old white, pleasant, well-educated, married female, mother of three children, with family history of hypercholesterolemia (father had aortic valve stenosis, and an aunt had aortic stenosis and coronary artery syndrome, and both had arcus senilis and xanthelesma). She was born, raised, and educated in Lebanon. Her aunt and uncle were also my patients but were not included in the study. I had referred the patient to a specialist to evaluate her hypercholesterolemia, following which she and her family moved to California. Her laboratory data, I believe, were reported in the published paper noted above.

Medically she was under the care of a local private physician. Her main complaint was exertional angina and chest tightness, making her short of breath on walking twenty to twenty-five yards, which abated with rest. She could also resume her walk at a slower pace with no further problems, and that is how she would do her daily walking exercise. She was being managed on a special low fat, low cholesterol diet without any other special medications. On examination, her blood pressure was 128/78 mmHg. Radial pulse was 74 bpm with a plateau upstroke. Neurological exam including orientation and cognizant function, sensory and motor and reflexes were intact.

The main findings were in the cardiovascular exam and the skin and tendons. Her skin was pale. Head and EENT exam revealed xanthelesma and arcus senilis; no lipid fundic emboli; otherwise, unremarkable. A systolic bruit was noted at the base of the cardia and neck transmitted from the base of the heart. Lungs were clear. Left ventricular heave was present. S1 and S2 were in regular sinus rhythm. Grade 4/6 midsystolic diamond-shaped murmur heard best over the base and aortic area, and transmitted to the base of the neck, accompanied by a systolic thrill.

The murmur ended beyond P2 indicating paradoxical split-second heart sound and A2 was diminished. Peripheral pulses were diminished. There was no hepato-splenomegaly or ascites or ankle edema.

Yellowish colored exanthema of Achilles tendons bilaterally. The ECG showed regular sinus rhythm with a rate of 76 bpm PR 0.16, QRS .08, left axis deviation, and depressed ST-T wave change in Ll, L2, V2–V6, consistent with coronary artery disease ischemia and/or left ventricular hypertrophy. Further, she needed to undergo 2-D echo (Doppler 2 D echo was not yet available) and lipid profile, as well as left-heart catheterization with coronary angiography. All of these studies were to be done with a referral to a university medical center, but were refused by the patient due to lack of medical insurance, in spite of the fact that I carefully explained the importance of going through with my recommendation.

In 1987, some twenty-five years after the initial diagnosis, the patient was admitted to a tertiary care medical center abroad for diagnosis and workup for possible cardiac surgery treatment for her coronary artery syndrome. Later, though I was not aware of her whereabouts, I received a surgical pathology report (shown on next page). The pathology diagnosis was severe atherosclerotic obstructive lesions of the two major coronaries with (aortic valve disease).

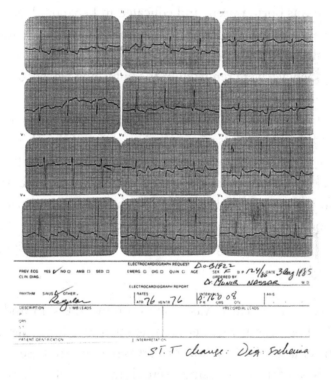

Shown above is an EKG of patient. Besides the effect of the ST-T wave changes noted,
the full interpretation is also suggestive of left ventricular hypertrophy.

The ascending aorta was extensively calcific, the calcification involving the aortic valve to a great extent, the aortic ring and the coronary ostea. The intima of this portion of the ascending aorta consisted of one plaque of bone involving the two coronary ostea with nodules in the region of the left coronary artery and the right coronary ostium.

Notes:

- The aortic valve calcification was extensive and involved the aortic ring. The very proximal portion of the ascending aorta could hardly admit the tip of a no. 17 Hegar dilator.
- The coronary vessels had a patent distal tree but the vessels looked atherosclerotic in their entirety.
- The right coronary ostium could not be visualized because of severe calcification, and could not be canulated because of the same.
- The left coronary ostium was covered by a nodule of calcific and could not be canulated. (Reference medical record, Departments of Pathology and Surgery, and the records room of the hospital.)
- On September 16, 2003, I submitted the patient's history, exam findings, and course, in abstract form, titled "A New Etiologic Factor for Aortic Stenosis: Relationship to Familial Hypercholesterolemia," to the American College of Cardiology for presentation at its annual meeting. The abstract was rejected for publication, despite the fact that the pathologic vascular endothelium lesion for aortic valvular stenosis with lipid and calcium deposits and foam cell formation is not documented in familial hypercholesterolemia, as was demonstrated in this patient. Though the etiology of aortic valve stenosis is obscure in the medical literature in this particular condition, it certainly deserves reporting for research. The above narrative is a summary of the abstract that was not published.

Study on a Missed Auscultatory Murmur in Rheumatic Pure Mitral Stenosis in Normal Sinus Rhythm

Introduction: This is a comparative study between the cardiologist's expert auscultatory diagnosis of rheumatic mitral stenosis and the surgeon's assessment of the stenotic valve commissurotomy in 157 patients out of 320 patients evaluated at the American University Medical Center from 1954–1967, and prior to echocardiography availability. Results: out of 320 rheumatic heart disease patients, 157 were found to have "pure" mitral valve stenosis by the same cardiologist. Evaluation included complete cardiovascular exam with ECG; cardiac series roentgenograms, left and right heart catheterization. with mitral valve area calculations, and phonocardiography. Classical auscultatory findings of diastolic rumble murmur of mitral stenosis and its components were present in all 157 patients. Sixty were males (38 percent), and ninety-seven (62 percent) were females. Age limits were twelve to fifty-six years. Fifty-one patients were Class II, eighty-eight were Class III, and eighteen were Class IV (New York Heart Association Classification). Pre-op: sixty-three were in (AF) atrial fibrillation, and of the ninety-three in normal sinus rhythm, twenty-six went into AF post-op. At surgery, all of the patients with regular sinus rhythm had "fish mouth" fused mitral leaflets and some with calcium deposits. The (same) surgeon's examining finger of the mitral valve noted invariably a whiff of regurgitant blood in systole that was not detected by auscultation in the pre-op evaluation. Conclusion: the whiff of systolic blood of "pure" mitral stenosis diastolic murmur is difficult to document clinically, though it may not be hemodynamically significant; this demonstrates proof of the accuracy of cardiac auscultation.

SECTION 2: My Research Experience in the USA

A Physician before the Time of Doctor William Harvey

The work of Dr. William Harvey (1578–1657) at Cambridge and Padua Universities established our current anatomical understanding of the systemic circulation of the blood. This dispelled sixteen centuries of anatomical ambiguities and conjecture portrayed by Galen in the second century, and follower Michael Servatus in the fourteenth century, but with one exception: the work of one Arab physician, Ibn An Nafis, who was born in Damascus, Syria, in the thirteenth century and was the dean of the Mansury Hospital in Cairo, Egypt. Today, Ibn An Nafis, though a much less recognized figure than Harvey, was the discoverer of the lesser circulation of the blood more than two hundred years prior to the work of Dr. William Harvey.[40, 41, 42]

This was documented in his *Commentary on the Canon of Ibn Sina*, another famous physician, philosopher, and astronomer, well-known all over the Arab world. Indeed it may be stated that Ibn An Nafis's work was a forgotten chapter in the history of the documented discovery of the circulation of the blood; namely, the pulmonary circulation.[43, 44]

Historical Discoveries and Perspectives

Prior to Galen, and in the Alexandrian School, Erasistratus expounded the belief that the spirit of the body was in empty arteries and in the left side of the heart.[45] Even today, people carry belief in the notion that the soul is in the heart. His main contribution was probably based on the remarkable insight of his teacher, Herophylos, who postulated that, in essence, there are two systems in the body. One system is that of the circulation of blood and that arteries are

---

40   William Harvey, "The Circulation of the Blood," trans., K. Franklin, *Everyman's Library* (Dutton, New York, 1966), v–xi, 1–113.

41   A. C. Cournand, "Air and Blood," *Circulation of the Blood; Men and Ideas*, eds., A. P. Fishman and D. W. Richards (New York: Oxford University Press, Inc., 1964), 9–18.

42   S. I. Haddad and A. A. Khairallah, "A Forgotten Chapter in the History of the Circulation of the Blood," *Annals of Surgery*, 104 (1936): 1–8. This is included in *Complete Works: Dr. Sami I. Haddad: History of Arab Medicine* (Beirut, Lebanon, 1975).

43   Ibid.

44   Mounir E. Nassar, "Arabian Medicine in the Middle Ages," *Journal of the Royal Society of Medicine* 77 (5) (1984): 438.

45   S. I. Haddad and A. A. Khairallah, "A Forgotten Chapter in the History of the Circulation of the Blood," *Annals of Surgery*, 104 (1936): 1–8. This is included in *Complete Works: Dr. Sami I. Haddad: History of Arab Medicine* (Beirut, Lebanon, 1975).

ten times thicker than veins and that heart "pulsations" are transmitted to the arteries with blood, and that in death the arteries are empty. The other system is breathing: absorption of fresh air and its elimination.[46] Erasistratus emphasized that there are two systems: circulation and breathing.

Two Centuries Later: Galen of Pergamon

Undoubtedly, Galen studied the work of predecessors and discredited them. He built what is known today as the "Galenic system of motion of the blood and air."[47] Though its contents are in error, it is still referred to as a milestone in the attempt of early physicians to understand the anatomy and physiology of the circulation of the blood.

Briefly stated, Galen refuted the notion that arteries are empty and showed that if one punctures an artery of a living mammal, blood is seen pouring out. However, he failed to understand pulmonary circulation and breathing. He stated that blood in the right side of the heart (right ventricle) passed through unseen pores to the left side of the heart, where it mixed with air and that constituted a spirit that was dispensed to the rest of the body.[48] Furthermore, he taught that a small amount of the blood from the left side returned backwards to the lungs to be cleared from its impurities. In addition, a small amount of right-side blood went through the vena arteriosus, to the arteriosus venosa, and to the left side of the heart. This shows the reader that, nevertheless, Galen had an obscure notion of the mysterious workings of pulmonary circulation, though the idea of a reflux is quite absurd.

The Thirteenth-Century Physician, Ibn An Nafis: a Mystery Unraveled

Serendipity may be a factor in the discovery of relevant facts in science. Looking closely at what is going to be narrated here may just fit the discovery of who was the discoverer of pulmonary circulation.

There lived in the thirteenth century a well-known Arab physician by the name of Ibn An Nafis (born in Damascus in 1210), who after completing his medical, philosophical, and religious studies, moved to Cairo, Egypt, and became the dean of the Mansury Hospital, where he also practiced medicine. He was a scholar in Islamic canon law, and a learned traditionalist in the Moslem way of life. Of the several medical volumes he authored, three will be mentioned.

---

46   William Harvey, "The Circulation of the Blood," trans., K. Franklin, *Everyman's Library* (New York: Dutton, 1966): v–xi, 1–113.

47   A. C. Cournand, "Air and Blood," *Circulation of the Blood; Men and Ideas*, eds. A. P. Fishman and D. W. Richards (New York: Oxford University Press, Inc., 1964), 9–18.

48   S. I. Haddad and A. A. Khairallah, "A Forgotten Chapter in the History of the Circulation of the Blood," *Annals of Surgery*, 104 (1936): 1–8. This is included in *Complete Works: Dr. Sami I. Haddad: History of Arab Medicine* (Beirut, Lebanon, 1975).

The first is *Al Mujaz*, which discussed the "perfect man" (it is similarly compared to progress in molecular and genetic medicine today).

The second is *Ash Shamil* (inclusive), a three-hundred-volume medical encyclopedia, of which Ibn Nafis completed eighty volumes.

Last, but not least, is his *Commentary on the Canon of Ibn Sina*, in which is found the description of the anatomy of the pulmonary circulation of the blood. It must be stated at the outset that human anatomical dissection was forbidden in Islamic law, and, from what Ibn Nafis stated himself, he adhered to it.[49] Ibn An Nafis's knowledge and his accurate anatomical description of the pulmonary circulation may have come from animal sources.

The *Commentary on the Canon of Ibn Sina* was discovered by chance in 1922 by an Egyptian medical student, Muhyi Din At Tatawi, at the Prussian Library. In 1924, Dr. Muhyi Din At Tatawi published his thesis in defense for his bachelor degree of medicine from the University of Freiburg in Brisgau.[50] It was then, and only then, that Western medicine was introduced to this important medical discovery, antedating the established work of Dr. William Harvey.

According to several scholars, Ibn Sina, born in Bukhara, was during his lifetime known by the title "Al Mu'allimuth Thani" (Arabic translation: the second teacher; Aristotle being the first). His *Qanun* or *Canon* consisted of 1,500 pages of medical knowledge, philosophy, and poetry. Though he was of Persian descent, he wrote his works in Arabic. He was revered as one of the brightest scholars of the time. It is of no surprise to note that Drs. William Osler and Harvey Cushing, and Professor Phillip Hitti were interested in Ibn Sina's life (980–1037) and work based on Greek knowledge and Galen's theory of the circulation of the blood.[51]

This *Commentary* by Ibn An Nafis refuted Galen's theory of pores in the interventricular septum, a mistake that was considered to be true for several centuries, well into the Middle Ages, bypassing Ibn An Nafis's work, until the time of Michael Servatus, and later Dr. William Harvey, where again Galen's theories were challenged and discarded. However, the *Commentary* of Ibn An Nafis remained in obscurity without being referred to. The reasons for such ambiguity will be discussed shortly.

Ibn An Nafis also described the anatomy of the lung in the following translation from Arabic into English (excerpt) by Drs. Sami Haddad and A. A. Khairallah.

---

49   Ibid.

50   A. C. Cournand, "Air and Blood," *Circulation of the Blood; Men and Ideas*, eds., A. P. Fishman and D. W. Richards (New York: Oxford University Press, Inc., 1964): 9–18.

51   S. I. Haddad and A. A. Khairallah, "A Forgotten Chapter in the History of the Circulation of the Blood," *Annals of Surgery*, 104 (1936): 1–8. This is included in *Complete Works: Dr. Sami I. Haddad: History of Arab Medicine* (Beirut, Lebanon, 1975).

The lung is composed of parts, one of which is the bronchi, the second the branches of the arteria venosa and the third the branches of the vena arteriosa, and all of these are connected by loose porous flesh …The need of the lung for the vena arteriosa is to transport to it the blood that has been thinned and warmed in the heart, so that what seeps through the pores of the branches of this vessel into the alveoli of the lung may mix with what there is of air therein and combine with it, the resultant composite becoming fit to be spirit when this mixing takes place in the left cavity of the heart. The mixture is carried to the left cavity by the arteria venosa.[52]

In another excerpt, he writes, "The vessel (vena arteriosa) carries back these things to the lung to be discharged with the returning breath (expiration)."

The Absence of the Commentary of Ibn An Nafis on the Anatomy of the Canon of Ibn Sina, from the Thirteenth to the Twentieth Century

This absence has baffled many scholars and remains a mystery that few historians have been able to even conjecture about as to what actually happened.

It is not, however, beyond certain known facts that point to the following scenario:

Two persons by the name of Andreas Alpagos and Paulos Alpagos lived in the Arab world for thirty years. They came to know the Arabic language, and they may have translated the *Commentary* and returned with it to Padua around 1530.

In that same period of time, there emerged an anti-Galen teaching, more in line with what scholars believe to be the anatomy of the pulmonary circulation. The problem with this scenario is that the *Commentary* was never recovered at the Padua School.[53]

Concluding Remarks

In any event, it is well known that Arab scholars preserved Greek and Roman cultures and combined them with Arab discoveries and thought on philosophy, medicine, algebra, and astronomy through the dark Middle Ages. It would not be out of context to theorize that the manuscript of Ibn An Nafis, along with many others, was translated by European scholars into Latin and Germanic languages, the likes of Gerard of Cremona and Albertus Magnus. It is not surprising, therefore, that the manuscript of Ibn An Nafis was discovered at the Prussian library in 1922.

---

52   Ibid.

53   A. C. Cournand, "Air and Blood," *Circulation of the Blood. Men and Ideas*, eds., A. P. Fishman and D. W. Richards (New York: Oxford University Press, Inc., 1964), 9–18.

A more scholarly question to ponder is whether Dr. William Harvey was aware of it or not when he was at Padua University in 1602. He was conferred upon a second doctor of medicine degree by Count Sigismund with witnesses (Drs. Fox and Lister).

It appears then that Dr. Harvey was unaware of the manuscript of Ibn An Nafis on the anatomy of the lesser circulation of the blood, since obviously the manuscript was never located or found at Padua University. Some scholars are still pondering, though, why it took Dr. William Harvey fourteen years after he left Padua for England to declare publicly his findings on the motion of the heart and the circulation of the blood.

Letter from Munir Nassar to the JRSM

From Dr. Munir E. Nassar, Albion, New York, USA

Dear Sir,

As a student of the history of medicine, I was interested to read the excellent paper by Shanks and Al-Kalai (January *Journal*, p. 60). With your permission, I would like to mention some pertinent references not included in their paper.

The first is the editorial by Dr. William Shuman (1927) presenting letters by Dr. M. Sa'eed, Dr. F. I. Shatara, and Dr. P. Hitti expounding the life and works of Avicenna and of the interest of Sir William Osler and Dr. Harvey Cushing in Avicenna's life and work.

In their paper, Shanks and Al-Kalai do not go beyond Avicenna's period to the thirteenth century, which was a period well-recognized by Arab physicians as a forgotten chapter in the history of Arabic medicine. In this connection there are two papers (Haddad 1936, Bittar 1955) that expound the discovery of the lesser circulation of the blood by Ibn Nafis. In his *Commentary on the Anatomy of Avicenna's Canon*, he clearly refuted Galen's theory of interventricular pores and described for the first time the lesser circulation and oxygenation of venous blood in the lung.

Finally there is Cournand's (1964) chapter "Air & Blood" in *Circulation of the Blood: Men and Ideas*. This makes fascinating reading on the subject and of the Greek, Persian, Arab, British, European, and US contributions to medicine.

Yours truly,

Munir E. Nassar
4 February 1984

References cited in my letter to the editor of JRSM are noted here.

- E. E. Bittar, MD thesis, (Yale University, 1955)
- A. C. Cournand in: *Circulation of the Blood: Men and Ideas*, eds., D. W. Richards and A. P. Fishman (New York: Oxford University Press, 1964)
- S. I. Haddad, *Muqtataf Journal* 89 (1936): 264
- W. Shuman, "Bulletin of the Los Angeles Medical Association," 57 (1927): 413–442

My research activity at Columbia University College of Physicians and Surgeons Cardiorespiratory Laboratory included contributions and assisting in three major works. First, the determination of the water space of the lung in dogs (normal value 3.5 ml/kg on average) and as a corollary, I suggested to study its application to lung blood vessels congestion versus lung edema to the principal investigators. Drs. O. Robert Levine, Robert B. Mellins, Mounir E. Nassar, and Alfred P. Fishman measured the abnormal changes of lung function in the congested lungs-edema of forty-one normal, anesthetized dogs. No reliable clinical criteria (rales. chest roentgenograms, and tidal volume) was noted differentiating lung congestion from edema. However, blood volume determination and comparing it to determination of the water space content at autopsy proved a reliable way experimentally to differentiate lung congestion from lung edema. The water space content was a constant 50 percent of the value of the total water content; hence a value of 6.0 ml/kg predicted lung edema at autopsy.

References:

- Presented at the Fifty-Sixth Annual Meeting of the American Society of Clinical Investigation, Atlantic City; May 4, 1964; p. 70.
- R. O. Levine, R. B. Mellins, and A. P. Fishman, "Quantitative Assessment of Pulmonary Edema," *Circulation Research*, XVII (November 1965): 414–426.

Dr. H. Yacoubian gave me permission to work on his unpublished paper. I took the opinion of my mentor, Dr. Dickinson W. Richards of Columbia University, who suggested a few modifications, which I implemented.

The study was on lung compliance on twenty-seven patients with predominantly mitral valve stenosis, on whom I had performed right heart catheterization, under the supervision of Dr. G. A. Rubeiz. The collected data was work on abnormal lung function carried over from my experience at the Cardiorespiratory Laboratory at Columbia University when I was assisting in the work on water space of the lung.

The lung compliance was markedly abnormal in lung edema in those patients. The conclusions from this study were that the lung compliance was inversely related to the mean capillary wedge pressure, and the higher the wedge pressure, the worse was the compliance, and the greater the increase in lung resistance to normal breathing. A new concept became evident: Degrees of dyspnea correlates better with increased total lung tissue resistance.

The Quantitative Assessment of Pulmonary Edema. O. ROBERT LEVINE, ROBERT B. MELLINS, MOUNIR E. NASSAR, AND ALFRED P. FISHMAN,* New York, N. Y.

In the intact animal or man, the degree of pulmonary edema is generally assessed by clinical and radiographic criteria. In this study, the degree of pulmonary edema was quantified by determining the interstitial water space of the lung (ISF) and the mechanics of breathing in dogs with graded degrees of pulmonary venous congestion. Pulmonary venous return was obstructed by inflating a balloon in the left atrium of anesthetized dogs followed by saline hemodilution. The ISF was determined from simultaneous T-1824 and tritiated water dilution curves; the results were compared with the water content of the lungs at autopsy. The forces responsible for formation of pulmonary edema were estimated from direct measurements of pulmonary arterial, left atrial, and oncotic pressures. In 33 dogs, control measurements of ISF ranged from 1.73 to 4.76 ml per kg (mean, 3.48 ml per kg; SD $\pm$ 0.22 ml per kg), and the pulmonary arterial-aortic arch blood volume (PBV) ranged from 11.5 to 17.3 ml per kg (mean, 15.2 ml per kg; SD $\pm$ 2.8 ml per kg). Balloon inflation and hemodilution resulted in pulmonary congestion in all 33 dogs; in 22 of these, there was also an increase in the ISF of 1 to 9 ml per kg. The ISF correlated significantly with lung weight and the moisture content of the lungs at autopsy. Pulmonary compliance and air flow resistance were also determined in eight dogs with pulmonary congestion. In those with normal ISF, compliance fell by 20 to 30%. In those with an expanded ISF (by 2.7 to 3.2 ml per kg) pulmonary compliance fell by 60 to 80%. Air flow resistance remained within normal limits in both groups. These data indicate that *1)* measurement of ISF distinguishes reliably between pulmonary congestion and edema and *2)* the effect of pulmonary congestion and edema on pulmonary compliance is quantitatively different.

My second research experience at the Cardiorespiratory Laboratory of Columbia University Presbyterian Hospital in New York, NY, involved producing and studying abnormal respiratory patterns in anesthetized intubated dogs. This included the recording of induced apnea followed by hyperventilation, using small doses of Pentothal, which was injected intravenously. I thought about how to translate this to treatment of sleep apnea at the clinical level, perhaps with the electronic manufacturing of a respiratory pacemaker.

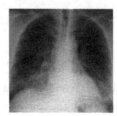

Referring to the above chest X-ray:

- Shows site of pneumotachograph encircling the chest wall of the patient above the right and left diaphragm.
- Two-way sensing electric probes inserted into the right and left diaphragm to stimulate the right and left diaphragm simultaneously with the same voltage as the phrenic nerves stimulating the diaphragm.

Electronic pacemaker with oscilloscope showing hyperventilation, then a period of ten seconds or more apnea, and then hyperventilation detected by the electronic pacemaker, which subsequently sends a stimulus impulse to the diaphragm to abort the apnea.

My third research experience at Columbia University Cardiorespiratory Laboratory and at St. Luke's Hospital was my assignment to study the mechanism of oscillations of the blood pressure. This problem was resolved using digoxin injected intravenously to induce Mobitz type 1 second-degree heart block and/or interference dissociation in anesthetized dogs. The recorded simultaneous EKG and blood pressure results clearly showed oscillations of the blood pressure with highest systolic value when the P-R interval was properly timed prior to the QRS on its sequence as shown in the EKG tracing. Hence I completed my required fellowship assigned project at the Cardiorespiratory Lab, Columbia University College of Physicians and Surgeons, NY, NY. This study was partly concluded at the Experimental Cardiac Lab at Columbia University, St. Luke's Hospital in NY, NY, under the direction of Dr. Robert B. Case.

Graph 1. Control: Respirations and Blood Pressure Waves

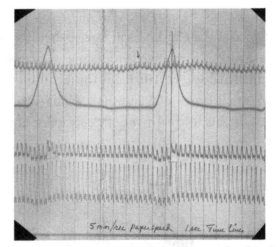

Graph 1 shows first the EKG above, second, respiration, third, pulmonary artery pressure mmHg, and the bottom of the tracing is the FA pressure mmHg.

Graph 2. Oscillations of the Femoral Artery Pressure of Anesthetized Dog Secondary to IV Digoxin.

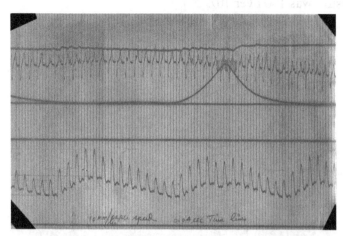

The top of Graph 2 shows EKG Interference Dissociation Auricular Rate 300/min, Ventricular Rate 350/min. Below it is the Respirations graph, and below that, is the Femoral Artery Pressure, varying between 180-140 mmHg systolic to 137-107 mmHg diastolic.

Graph 3. Oscillations of the Femoral and Pulmonary Artery Pressure of Anesthetized Dog Secondary to IV Digoxin.

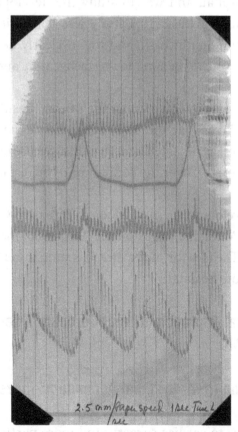

The top of Graph 3 shows the EKG, below it, respirations. Again, Oscillations of the Femoral Artery, Systolic and Diastolic Pressure, 180-140 over 137-107.

Graph 4. Shows the EKG rhythm interference dissociation and oscillations of the femoral artery pressure at 10 mm paper speed per second and the timelines are .04 seconds. The femoral artery pressure was 180 over 107.

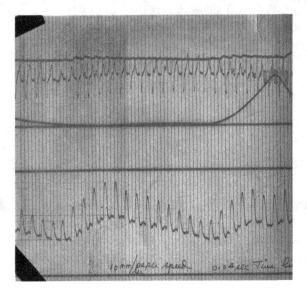

My fourth research experience was a purely clinical one at the cardiac monitoring unit of Columbia-Presbyterian Hospital, and was to study the development of cardiac arrest on patients with coronary cardiac disease. This study was done with the lead investigators of Drs. Richard Stock, Hamilton Southworth, and me. It clearly demonstrated the premature ventricular beat on the T wave phenomenon causing tachycardia and/or ventricular fibrillation.

This clinical research study was presented under the title of "Results of a Cardiac Monitoring Unit in Treating Cardiac Arrest" at the 38th Scientific Session of the American Heart Association, October 1965. It may be stated here that this was the impetus for the development of "cardiac" intensive care units all over the country and the rest of the world.

I was the motivator for developing the first Medical Intensive Care Unit at the Methodist Hospital, Baylor College of Medicine, Houston, in 1959–1960, for the treatment of complex, serious medical conditions. The idea for such a unit was similar to Dr. M. E. Debakey's surgical intensive care unit at the same hospital.

The Invention for a Surgical Approach to Treat Coronary Artery Syndromes: the Inventor, Mounir Nassar, MD

Background of the Invention (refer to "Final Addendum" for references)

The present invention relates to cardiac surgery, and more particularly relates to a surgical technique of using an auricular appendage graft to augment areas of weakened heart muscle.

It applies to patients with acute or chronic coronary artery syndromes who have or have not undergone CABG or PCI and are Class I-II cardiacs according to the New York American Heart Association Classification. The surgical approach is to prevent further cardiac heart failure deterioration. Furthermore, the patients are being treated medically for early signs and symptoms of heart failure.

Congestive heart failure occurs when the heart fails to deliver a sufficient output of blood to meet the metabolic requirements of the organs and tissues of the body. Its manifestations include a lower blood pressure resulting in poor perfusion of tissues, which may result in conditions such as dyspnea, orthopnea, and nocturnal paroxysmal dyspnea secondary to lung fluid congestion-edema, high jugular venous pressure, renal insufficiency, and peripheral pitting edema. A type of congestive heart failure includes systolic dysfunction due to impaired myocardial contraction leading to left ventricular failure. There are many causes of congestive heart failure including hypertension, acute and chronic coronary artery syndromes, myocardial infarction, and valvular aortic and mitral valve disease being the common causes of low ejection fraction below 40 percent.

The other type of congestive heart failure is diastolic dysfunction, manifested by nonpliable, stiff left ventricle resulting in low blood pressure with "normal" ejection fraction. Both types of congestive heart failure described above may occur simultaneously in the same patient.

Summary of the Invention

The present invention describes and claims a treatment for congestive heart failure due to acute or chronic coronary artery syndromes with myocardial infarction, or absence of ST change of myocardial infarction. Other indications are: (1) prior coronary artery bypass graft, (2) percutaneous coronary stent failure. All may result in congestive heart failure. The inventive technique involves surgically transplanting the right or left auricular appendage of the heart to the damaged weakened area of the diseased myocardium. (It is important to preserve the venae cavae and the sinoatrial node on the right and pulmonary veins on the left, depending on which auricular appendage is used.) A team of cardiothoracic surgeon(s) and cardiologist(s) is required. Cardiac echoes and cardiac output will be measured pre- and post-op and followed up with chest X-ray, electrocardiogram, and cardiac echoes with physical therapy for several months. This procedure may be perfected in experiments on animals with induced coronary artery blockage in dogs, cats, sheep, etc., to verify its applicability to humans with coronary artery syndromes.

Brief Description of the Drawing

Figure 1. A view of a human heart (from "Cardiac Catheterization" published by the American Heart Association, copyright 1998, 1995 by Health Trend Publishing, Menlo Park, CA) modified to show the auricular appendages and blockage or narrowing of one or another coronary artery.

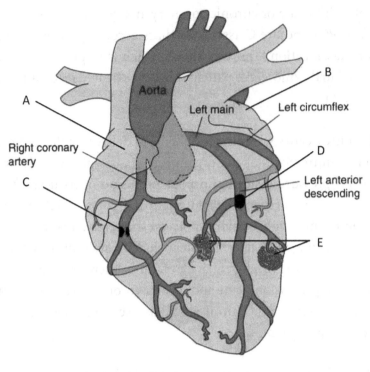

The Coronary Arteries

The two left coronary arteries (left anterior descending and left circumflex) supply blood to the front, left side, and back of the heart. The right coronary artery supplies blood to the bottom, right side, and back of the heart.

A. The right atrial appendage, part of the right atrium
B. The left atrial appendage, part of the left atrium
C. Narrowing of right coronary artery due to atherosclerosis or plaque
D. Complete blockage of left anterior descending artery
E. Necrotic or damaged myocardial area from blocked left anterior descending coronary artery; schematic representation of areas of infarc which in actuality may be larger than what is portrayed

Using special surgical technique, with preservation of the right or left atrium, transplanting the appendage (A) of either atria to the damaged muscle (E) treating the infarced area where the transplant will take over and produce circulation and strengthen the damaged muscle area, thus preventing, in the long run, congestive heart failure. The same surgical technique can be applied for symptomatic narrowing of the right anterior coronary artery, improving the circulation and resolving the angina or acute coronary heart syndrome.

This aforementioned approach to remedy myocardial ischemia and/or myocardial necrosis with production of collateral circulation is also applicable to coronary balloon angioplasty treatment with or without stenting failure (including elution stents) or to coronary artery bypass graft failure. In addition, on theoretical implications the auricular appendage transplant can be used at the time of coronary artery bypass graft surgery.

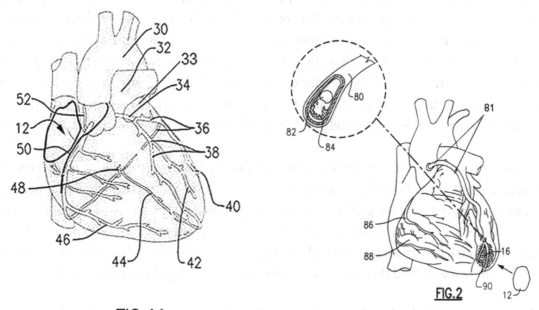

FIG.1A

Figures 1A and 2 above are examples of myocardial infarction with cabbage, and an atrial appendage applied to the dying cardiac muscle. Please note that other conditions causing myocardial infarction are not illustrated here but are included in the text.

Figure 1A Legend

12	right atrium with auricle appendage
30	aortic arch
32	pulmonary artery
33	left atrium with appendage
34	left coronary artery
36	circumflex branch of left coronary artery
38	left anterior descending coronary artery
40	continuation of left circumflex branch
42	lateral diagonal branch
44	branch of right coronary artery
46	branch of right coronary artery
48	branch of right coronary artery
50	right coronary artery
52	right coronary artery

Figure 2 Legend

12	left atrial appendage patch
16	dying cardiac muscle
80	left anterior descending blockage
81	bypass artery graft from aorta
82	blood clot
84	cholesterol plaque
86	coronary arteries
88	healthy muscle
90	dying cardiac muscle

Detailed Description

Referring now to the drawing, there is seen in the figure a human heart, which includes right and left auricle appendages that are extensions of the main right and left atrium, respectively. Figure 1 is a view of the heart showing a blocked left anterior descending artery with infarction of muscle area of the heart. If the bypass graft segment gets blocked in the future, the patient may have a second heart attack. If the blockage is gradual, the area of cardiac muscle supplied by the graft may start to fail to contract well and heart failure may ensue. A balloon angioplasty may be inserted into a blocked coronary artery and inflated to relieve obstruction in the coronary artery. A stent can then be inserted to keep the vessel open, although stents are also known to occasionally fail.

According to the present invention, either of the auricular appendages is excised and transplanted onto the affected area in the manner of a graft. Since the auricular appendages are muscular tissue, once the graft has taken hold, the auricular tissue will assist the cardiac muscle in this area to restore normal pumping action to the heart. It is expected that the transplanted auricular appendage will take as a graft, provide collateral circulation to the areas affected, and restore blood flow and also strengthen the damaged myocardial wall.

An Invention of a Method and Apparatus for Treating Sleep Apnea and/or Weaning a Patient off a Ventilator: the Inventor, Mounir Nassar, MD

Background of the Invention

The present invention relates to treatment of sleep apnea, and more particularly relates to a treatment using a special sensor/activator pacemaker.

The definition of sleep apnea is cessation of respiratory tidal volume during sleep for ten seconds or longer with hardly any thoracic/chest bellows movements in humans. Causes are well-documented in standard medical texts and range from micro- or macrognathia, hypothyroidism, anatomical upper airway obstruction, COPD, upper airway restriction, obesity, congestive heart failure, stroke, and respiratory depressant drugs. A special type of apnea was described by Cheyne and Stokes due to anoxia secondary to low PO_2 of high altitude. Breathing was controlled by the medulla chemoreceptor centers receiving afferent impulses from the vagus and glossopharyngeal nerve reacting to send efferent impulses to diaphragms and intercostals muscles via phrenic and spinal nerves causing inspiration and passive expiration breathing. Chemoreceptors in the medulla detect changes in CO_2 and pH of cerebrospinal fluid (CSF) to initiate nerve impulses. The central nervous system cortex may also take voluntary control over the medulla for breathing. Chemoreceptors in carotid bodies of aortic arch detect decrease in the arterial PO_2 and O_2 saturation at a critical level to initiate breathing. Also the apneustic center in the vestibulari is important in stroke and in decerebrate rigidity lesions. Finally, there is the pnuemotaxic center in the pons also important in stroke

There are basically three classifications of sleep apnea: (1) CSA, central sleep apnea, or Cheyne Stokes; (2) OSA, obstructive sleep apnea, that may be seen in patients with COPD, for example; and (3) mixed, a combination of CSA and OSA. The basic neurological controls for breathing rate malfunction and fail to give the signal to inhale, causing the individual to miss one or more cycles of breathing.

The current popular treatment of sleep apnea includes using a CPAP (continuous positive air pressure) mask at night. If the cause is an obstruction in the mouth or throat, surgery may be required. While these treatments have met with some success, there remains a need for an improved method and apparatus for treating sleep apnea, particularly for those patients in which existing treatment modalities are not effective.

Summary of the Invention

The present invention addresses the above need by providing a unique, as termed herein, "sleep apnea pacemaker" apparatus and method for treating sleep apnea. In an embodiment of the invention, an ECG monitor may be attached to the sleeping patient to display dysrhythmia during sleep indicating sleep apnea. An oxygen pressure monitor is also attached to the patient. Hyperventilation is indicated when the blood oxygen saturation level is greater than about 96 percent and the oxygen pressure drops. Apnea is indicated when blood oxygen saturation level dips below about 85 percent for a period of at least ten seconds with a resultant rise in oxygen pressure. The patient attaches a pneumotachygraph (an apparatus for recording the rate of airflow to and from the lungs, i.e., the bellows action of the thorax) attached to the thorax immediately prior to sleep. The pneumotachygraph is attached to a gauge galvanometer and to an oscilloscope, which is wired to a pacemaker comprising two electrodes which are inserted in the patient's right and left diaphragm. The oscilloscope will detect sleep apnea and send an electric impulse to activate the diaphragm to contract and abort the apnea period.

Such a respiratory pacemaker may be useful to attempt to wean patients off mechanical ventilation apparatus.

Study Abstract on the Proof of Importance of Normally Timed Atrial Contraction to Cardiac Stroke Output and Blood Pressure in Anesthetized Dogs

Control/tracking number: 03-A-262106-ACC Activity: Abstract
Current date/time: 8/4/2002 12:36:25 p.m.

Proof of Importance of Normally Timed Atrial Contraction to Cardiac Stroke Output and Blood Pressure in Anesthetized Dogs

Munir E. Nassar, Robert B. Case, St. Luke's Hospital Experimental Cardiology Lab, New York, New York.

Introduction:

In studying intravenous (IV) digoxin toxicity in anesthetized dogs, and Wenkebach (Mobitz type 1), regularly recurring marked oscillations of the monitored blood pressure (BP) was recorded. The purpose of this study was to determine the effect of varying the timing of interval occurrence of atrial systole (PR interval on the ECG) and its effect on ventricular stroke output and blood pressure. Methods: Six mongrel dogs were anesthetized with IV Nembutal and intubated and mechanically ventilated. The femoral artery was canulated and attached to a BP gauge. ECG electrodes monitored rhythm. Second degree (Mobitz type l) was produced following IV digoxin (dose 3.5–4 mg) (in six out of ten dogs). Left ventricular stroke output for each systole (excluding coronary sinus flow) was measured using a flow meter around aortic root. Simultaneous measurements were made of pressure in left atrium, left ventricle, aorta, and airway. Results: When the PR interval fell below 0.01 seconds, left atrial pressure rose from an average 9.9 to 25.3 mmHg, and stroke output decreased from mean of 7.2 to 5.7 ml/beat, with a fall in aortic pressure on average to 179 from 197 at PR interval of 0.16 seconds. Conclusions: Normally timed atrial contraction is an important stabilizing influence on stroke output and BP. Otherwise oscillations in those parameters occurred with Mobitz type 1.

Other data collected:

Category (complete): clinical electrophysiology–supraventricular arrhythmias

Keywords (complete): atrial function, cardiac output, blood pressure

Additional (complete): The ALLHAT Collaborative Study and its clinical implications: "Antihypertenesive Lipid Lowering Treatment to Prevent Heart Attack." The study was conceived based on risk factors of hypertension and elevated cholesterol.

Aside from my clinical work as chief medical officer at the Veterans Affairs of Western New York, I had the opportunity to participate in the ALLHAT Study as chief collaborator for screening, examining, and enrolling qualified veterans of Western NY into the clinical randomized study.

The total number of enrolled patients from all over the VA centers in the United States was 33,387. The age of patients was fifty-five years and over with a mean age of sixty-seven years. Follow-up was over a five-year period.

Breakdown by gender and ethnic background:

53 percent were male
47 percent were female
Total 100 percent

35 percent were African American, 19 percent were Hispanics, and 46 percent were white Caucasian.

Of the total number of patients enrolled 36 percent were diabetic.

The study was published in *JAMA* 288 (2002): 2981–2991.

Conclusions of the study:

- For first approach to antihypertensive treatment was that thiazide type drugs were effective in low dose chlorthalidone 12.5 mg per day and adding a calcium channel blocker, amlodipine 5mg–10mg per day with a statin, lisinopril, was effective in controlling blood pressure below 139/89.
- Step 2—add an ace inhibitor.
- Step 3—hydralazine may be added for difficult, not well-controlled blood pressure, if required. For the hypertensive patients, 60 percent had a lowering of their blood pressure to below 140/90 mmHg.

SECTION 3: Epilogue: Evidence-Based Medicine and Epistemology—A Cautionary Tale for Physicians

Two basic concepts integral to the practice of medicine also are at the heart of the philosophical field of epistemology. The first is the concept of gathering scientific evidence; the second is the concept of experiencing perceived clinical symptoms in sick patients.

Epistemology is the study of the origin of knowledge. Philosophical arguments relating to the source of knowledge date back to the early Greeks. Plato refutes the theory that knowledge is derived from sensual perceptions, which can be vague and ambiguous. True knowledge, Plato believed, is related to concepts, such as 2+2=4.

Aristotle, on the other hand, was interested in the roles induction and deduction play in the ways we acquire knowledge. For example, we may assume that a figure we call John Doe is mortal, basing that assumption on our observation that all John Does born 140 years ago clearly are dead. This use of inductive reasoning offers a probability about longevity, while certainty about longevity requires a deductive process. The former opens new vistas of knowledge of mortality, whereas the latter is a closed case (adapted fromWhitehead).

Descartes (1596–1650) states that when an idea is clearly perceived in the mind, unaccompanied by doubts, that idea is true. He uses the now famous example, "Je pense, donc je suis." ("I think, therefore I am.") John Locke (1632–1704), on the other hand, relied on information provided by the senses as this sensual information is inscribed on our brains, a receptive organ that begins as a "tabula rasa," or blank page. The brain analyzes these inscripted, sense-derived experiences and formulates them into ideas. For David Hume (1711–1776), like Descartes, the existence of the physical world is within our minds, created by our sensual impressions. For this reason, Hume believed, it is difficult to prove its existence outside our minds.

Emanuel Kant (1724–1804) disagreed. For him, Descartes and Hume's position was flawed because of the absence of any experimental basis in their approach to epistemology. Kant's theory is that knowledge of the reality of the outside world is gained through experiences in spatial-time events. One's senses do not portray events in time; rather one's creative mind ties together perceived sensations from the outside world in a timely manner.

More recent epistemological theories are based on the work of Bertrand Russell (1872–1970) and A. N. Whitehead (1861–1947). They believed that knowledge of the physical world can be gained in abstract ways. Analysis of the relationship of objects in the physical world, such as their structure, establishes the reality of nature as existing outside our minds but explained by our minds.

Let's put aside this brief historical review and see how such concepts relate to the practice of evidence-based medicine. I draw here on two examples from my own practice.

Case 1: One day a thirty-seven-year-old man, whom I had not seen before, came to my office complaining of a markedly reduced exercise tolerance, dyspnea on mild exertion (such as walking level ten yards), and lower extremity edema of a few weeks' duration. Examination revealed a BP of 140/64, borderline sinus tachycardia, respiration rate of 24/min, elevated jugular venous pulse, and 12 cm of water above angle of Lewis.

The fellow was mentally alert, anxious, and oriented; his neurological exam was normal. He had bilateral basal rales, gallop rhythm, a grade 4/6 diastolic murmur over the aortic area radiating down the left sternal cardiac border, and a 36 systolic murmur at the base of the heart radiating to the base of the neck. There were no signs of embolic phenomena or elevated temperature.

My impression was that of major aortic regurgitation, with either associated stenosis or aortic aneurysm, and congestive cardiac failure, Class III NYHA Classification. My clinical impression (based on learned experience) was that the man had a dilated boot-shaped heart, with lung congestion and a dilated aortic root. Subsequent roentgenogram confirmed the lung congestion and dilated aortic root; an echo cardiogram confirmed the aortic regurgitation, aortic root aneurysm, and dilated left ventricle; and an echo cardiogram confirmed left ventricular hypertrophy and a normal sinus rhythm.

The physician in such a case need not wait to obtain other evidence (such as the result of syphilis serology and blood cultures to rule in or out infective endocarditis) to begin treatment. Indeed, treatment for heart failure should start immediately, with referral for urgent cardiac surgery to repair the damaged aortic value and aneurysm.

Case 2: Evidence-based medicine does have a place in cases where the patient has significant weight loss, fever of unclear origin, potential anemia, etc. But again, it's one's learned medical experience in such cases that comes first.

At one time, my practice abroad included a poor primitive rural area where the local hospital and laboratory closed their doors to business at 5:00 p.m. each day. Once, I was wakened around midnight and called to attend a sick patient at his home. The courier who summoned me stated that local doctors had seen the man, but that his health was not improving. Since I was on the faculty of medicine at the university, my opinion was sought. On examining the man, I found he had a low-grade fever of 38.5 OC, a bradycardic pulse of 58/min, frontal headache, mild abdominal pain, no signs of acute abdomen, a palpable spleen, and no skin rash.

My clinical diagnosis was typhoid fever. I gave the patient a chloramphenicol prescription and instructions on how to take the medicine, as well as advice on nutritious diet and sanitation. I instructed him to summon the laboratory as soon as possible for a confirmatory test for typhoid, to have his local doctor follow up on his condition, and to contact me if the need arose.

My point in linking the history of epistemology and these two clinical cases is this: learned and refined clinical experience often precedes evidence-based medicine. In fact, waiting for evidence-based medicine results before beginning treatment may place the patient at risk, especially those who have a GI bleed, developing endocarditis, or, as in the case of my rural patient, a potentially fatal infection.

Concluding remarks: This manuscript is a testimonial of the efforts of many physicians who brought clinical medical research up to par with the practice of medicine.

It is without question that the Faculty of Medicine of the American University of Beirut has had its shining moments in what I believe was its golden age (1920–1970) and the future remains to be written.

I would like to conclude with a plea. The efforts of the new generation of physicians should be directed to reestablishing the high stature of the practicing physician in society. One way to achieve such a standard is to curb the growth of the "business" of medicine. The practice of medicine is a calling to help cure patients from disease, not for the sole sake of material profit.

Mounir E. Nassar, MD, FACP
May 28, 2012

Further notation about the events of 1882 in the Department of Medicine of SPC:

Dr. Edwin Rufus Lewis, MD, from Harvard Medical School, was professor of chemistry and biology at the Syrian Protestant College. In 1882, he was relegated to deliver the commencement address to the graduating class. His title was "Knowledge, Science and Philosophy." In his address, he encouraged the graduates to continue to pursue knowledge and read about the discoveries of Robert Koch (discoverer of the Koch TB bacillus), Louis Pasteur and his discovery of infection as a cause of disease, and also Charles Darwin. The latter name produced a bad taste to the conservative professors of the faculty, Rev. Daniel Bliss, and the commission in New York, and it resulted in Dr. Lewis's dismissal.

This event split the medical department, with certain prominent support for Dr. Lewis from Dr. C. Van Dyck, who resigned from the department along with some students. [*MainGate* (Winter 2012): 43.]

Further explanation of Dr. Fawaz's synthesis of phosphocreatine:

Now going to the Department of Pharmacology and the published works of Dr. G. Fawaz, I would like to mention the following: the crowning achievement of his research was the synthesis of phosphocreatine. There are several chemicals and biochemical reactions involved with cardiac muscle relaxation and contraction. These include ionized Ca, Mg, Creatine Kinase, troponine 1 and C, ATPase and ATP and ADP that are involved in the separation and recombination of Actin-Myosin (actin and myosin). The energy propelling these biochemical reactions comes from ATP $\longleftrightarrow$ ADP with the catalyst phosphocreatine $\longleftrightarrow$ creatine and phosphate. Hypertensive cardiovascular disease, coronary artery syndromes, cardiomyopathies, valvular heart disease, and certain congenital heart disease compromise the "Starling Law of the Heart" mechanical forces, eventually impacting on the biochemical reactions of cardiac muscle relaxation and contraction, resulting in the complex problem of congestive heart failure. [Clive Rosendorf, et al., *Clinical Cardiovascular and Pulmonary Physiology* (New York: Raven Press, 1983), 36–37.] Such a textbook was excellent material for clinical research by clinicians.

This is a preliminary elucidation of the importance of phosphocreatine and may require additional information which is not the purpose of this work.

Mounir E. Nassar, MD, FACP
May 28, 2012

On the campus, the first medical building that housed the Medical Department was the first building on the right upon entering the Medical Gate. Later in the life of the AUB, at our time it housed the Social Science Department, and eventually it housed the School of Public Health. In 1929, with a small Rockefeller grant, the C. V. Cornelius Hall became a reality, and it housed the preclinical sciences, an amphitheater, and a medical library. In front of the hall, as decoration, a small walled pond with a beautiful flower garden completed the hall.

Dr. Post was not of the original medical faculty. He was appointed later.

It is important to state that the origin of the college (or university) began in Abeih. Later it moved to Beirut and was located in the Boutros Boustani building.

Dr. Farid S Haddad, in a forthcoming book titled, *Dr. George A. Fawaz* (in press), in chapter 32, discusses the work of Dr. Harris Graham on dengue: "Dr. Graham and abul' alrikab."

Rephrasing the statement on the crisis of 1882, it probably was not related to the pauicity of medical research by the faculty of SPC.

It is of importance to pay tribute to the contributions of Dr. Sami I. Haddad by listing them in detail. Besides the introduction of cystoscopy, Dr. Sami I. Haddad introduced to the Middle East the following:

- total radical laryngectomy for cancer of the larynx (Billroth's operation)
- surgical collapse therapy for pulmonary tubersulosis (415 cases)
- the earliest direct blood transfusion prior to the establishment of the blood banks
- a modification of Millin's retropubic prostatectomy with preservation of the urethra
- the use of local anesthesia for major operations such as amputation, bowel resection, cholecystectomy, hydatid cyst of lung, recurrent breast cancer, ovarian twist cyst, pyelolithotomy, strangulated umbilical hernia, thyroidectomy, tonsillectomy, ureterolithotomy
- cholecystectomy through a kidney lumbar approach

He even operated on himself.

Dr. Hitti is credited in the writing and publishing of the *English Arabic Dictionary*.

The bibliography of Dr. Farid S. Haddad deserves special mention. It consists of

- 1,570 published works, including 70 books;
- 704 written unpublished articles, all available in *Annotated and Illustrated Bibliography* (Rancho Palos Verdes: The Sami I. Haddad Memorial Library, 2007); and
- the "firsts" (407 original contributions) of Dr. Farid Sami Haddad found in *Harvest of a Lifetime* (Rancho Palos Verdes: The Sami I. Haddad Memorial Library, 2010).

A special experiment by Dr. Fouad Salim Haddad deserves mention; he wrote about "the first use of anesthesia in the chicken in Abeih."

Dr. Oliver should be included in the Department of ENT.

For the record, Dr. Charles A. Webster (Rev) wrote three papers: "Medical Notes," *Al Kulliyeh*, III (1912): 171–173; the second was about his visit to Egypt, *Al Kulliyeh* (1911): 165–169; and the third paper was "Some Experiences of a Happy Furlough," *Al Kulliyeh* (1914): 60–65. He also wrote a book on the ear.

This should include a complete bibliography of Dr. Sami I. Haddad of 295 items, 106 of which are articles (60 in English and 46 in Arabic). Also, he undertook 66 radio talks in Arabic and 17 books. Those items have been listed and analyzed in Dr. Farid S. Haddad's book, *A First-Class Man in Every Particular* on pages 215–228. For the interested reader, all the writings of Dr. Sami I. Haddad have been collectively republished in the following volumes:

- *History of Arab Medicine*, 1975
- *Arab Medicine and Islamic Hospitals*, (2003 Edition)
- *Surgical and Medical Articles*
- *Recent Advances in Medicine, Final Gleanings, History of the Arabic Script*, (2004 Edition)
- *The Orchard*, (2006 Edition)

It should be noted that the references above are in Arabic titles. However, for the sake of English readers, the titles are mentioned in English.

A correction is noted that *Almwjaz* and the *Perfect Man* are two separate books.

Another correction, The "Commentary on the Canon" should read "Commentary on the Anatomy of the Canon" (Sharh at Tasrih of Law in Medicine). Also, the "Commentary" was not discovered by chance, but Dr. Al Tatawi studied it for his thesis dissertation.

A clarification is that the Canon is a complete medical text. It has remained the Bible for medical students for over 1,000 years. It does not contain philosophy or poetry. Avecenna also wrote books on philosophy and one poetry book, *The Cantica*.

Two articles had published experiments on the feasibility of using bilateral atrial appendage grafts to (a) artificially produced coronary ischemia by ligation of a branch of the left anterior descending coronary artery in one series of anesthetized dogs, and (b) in another, removal of a small transmyocardial segment simulating myocardial infarction in a series of anesthetized dogs. Both series were compared to normal dogs with grafts, with a ten-week follow-up with good take of the grafts and good microscopic collateral circulation at autopsy. [Dr. Shapiroff and coworkers, *J Thoracic Surg.* (1951): 631–635.] The second reference, by Dr. T. Sakai and coworkers, used cultured atrial myocytes and transplanted those cells onto cryosurgically induced injury to the myocardium of rats with follow up after five weeks, with good take and improved myocardial function. [Dr. Sakai and coworkers, *Ann. of Thoracic Surg.* 68 (1999):2074–2080].

1. Rubeiz, G., and M. E. Nassar. "The Significance of the Post Extrasystolic T Wave Change. *Lebanese Medical Journal,* 14 (1961): 181–186.

2. Dagher, I. K., G. Rubeiz, M. E. Nassar, S. Nassif, H. Yacoubian, R. Tabbara, and J. L. Wilson. "Open Intracardiac Repair of Tetralogy of Fallot." *Leb. Med. J.* 17 (1964): 7–14.

3. Rubeiz, G., M. E. Nassar, and I. K. Dagher. "Study of the Right Atrial Pressure in Functional Tricuspid Regurgitation and Normal Sinus Rhythm." *Circulation* 30 (1964): 190–193.

4. Nassar, M.E. "The Intensive Care Unit." *Leb. Med. J.* 21 (1968): 209–291.

5. Mugrditchian, P., and M. E. Nassar. "Lung Function Norms of Lebanese Children and Adolescents." *Middle East J Anesthesiology* 2 (1970): 6–11.

6. Levine, O.R., R. B. Mellins, M. E. Nassar, and A. P. Fishman. "Quantitative Assessment of Pulmonary Edema." *J. Clinical Investigation* 43 (1964): 1294. Presented at the 56th Annual Meeting of the American Society of Clinical Investigation.

7. Stock, R., M. E. Nassar, H. J. Myers, and H. Southworth. "Results of a Cardiac Monitoring Unit in Treating Cardiac Arrest." *Circulation* 31 & 31 (supp. II) (1965): 203. Presented at the 38th Scientific Session of the American Heart Association, October 1965.

8. Nassar, M. E. "Unusual Physical Sign of Multiple Myeloma." *J Royal Society of Medicine* 76 (1983): 157–158 (case report).

9. Nassar, M. E. Letter to Editor: "U.S.F.M.G. and Their Board Scores." *N Engl J Med.* 298 (1986): 169.

10. Nassar, M. E. "Treatment of Respiratory Failure." *J Royal Society of Medicine* (July 1985).

11. Nassar, M. E. "Basic Life Support Manuscript." Work done at Shepard AFB Dept. of Medical Education ATC 1978.

12. Nassar, M. E. Letter to Editor: "Viagra, Latest Cardiovascular Drug." Response to editorial of Dr. Conti *Clin. Cardiol* 21 (1998): 616. Published January 1999: 22(1): 2.

13. Nassar, M. E. Electronic Rapid Response: "Changing Natural History of the Diagnosis of Congestive Heart Failure." *BMJ* 325 (September 3, 2002): 422–425.

14. Nassar, M. E. Electronic Rapid Response: "Changing Natural History of Congestive Heart Failure." *BMJ* (September 11, 2002).

15. Nassar, M. E. "Proof of Importance of Proper Timed Atrial Contraction to Stroke Output (Ventricular Systole) and Systolic Blood Pressure in Anesthetized Dogs." Abstract submitted to the ACC's 51st Annual Scientific Session 2002 (unpublished).

16. Nassar, M. E. "Rheumatic Heart Disease Mitral Stenosis in Lebanon." Abstract submitted to the ACC's 51st Annual Session 2002 (unpublished).

17. Nassar M. E. Electronic Rapid Response:"10-Minute Consultation: Dyspepsia." "Other causes of Dyspepsia." *BMJ* 322 (November 16, 2003):776.

18. Nassar, M. E. Electronic Rapid Response: "Additional Comments to 'ABC of Heart Failure.'" *BMJ* (January 1, 2000).

19. Nassar, M. E. Electronic Rapid Response: "Further Comments on 'Congestive Heart Failure.'" *BMJ* (May 9, 2000).

20. Nassar, M. E. Electronic Rapid Response: "B Blockers and 'Congestive Heart Failure." *BMJ* (May 5, 2000).

21. Nassar, M. E. Electronic Rapid Response: "Vaccination for N. Menningitides." *BMJ* (March 25, 2000).

22. Nassar, M. E. Electronic Rapid Response: "Prognosis in Heart Failure." *BMJ* (January 25, 2000).

23. Nassar, M. E. Electronic Rapid Response: "The Problem with Seven-Day Treatment of Group A Streptococcus Tonsillitis—Pharyngitis." *BMJ* (January 16, 2000).

24. Nassar, M. E. "Cancer Screening with the Use of Genetic Abnormality in Mitochondrial Cells from Body Fluids." *BMJ* (March 25, 2000).

25. Nassar, M. E. "Nurse Practitioners." *ACP-ASIM Observer* (1998): 18, P2.

26. Nassar, M. E. Electronic Rapid Response: "The C-Reactive Protein Revisited." *BMJ* (October 2000) and *BMJ* (January 9, 2001).

27. Nassar, M. E. Electronic Rapid Response to Editorial: A. Cilliers, "Treatment of Acute Rheumatic Fever," *BMJ* 327 (2003): 631–632. "Why Not Absolute Bed Rest for Acute Rheumatic Fever?" *BMJ* (Jamuary 10, 2004).

28. Nassar, M. E. To the Editor, *ACP Observer*: HIPAA Compliance, Problems, Errors, and Disclosures: Jan–Feb 2004. "Alerting Physicians to Ordered X-Rays or Lab Results due to Abnormal Results." Under consideration.

29. Nassar, M. E. "Appraisal of the US Healthcare System Revisited." Unpublished observations.

30. Nassar, M. E. "Treatment of Sleep Apnea of 10 Sec or More with Automatic Phrenic/ Diaphragmatic Electronic Pacemaker Stimulation." Work in progress; all rights reserved.

31. Nassar, M. E. "A Doctor's Research Experience." Copyright reserved.

32. Nassar, M. E. Letter to Editor: *Patient Care*, March 15, 2001: "Where Antibiotic Resistance Reigns." (Response to "Refining Empiric Prescribing of Antibiotics," January 30, 2001.) Note correction: fifth line, second paragraph to read "may" prescribe … instead of "must."

33. Nassar, M. E. Electronic Rapid Response: "Additional Risk Predictors of Morbidity and Mortality of Cardiovascular Disease in Adults." *BMJ* (July 18, 2001).

34. Nassar, M. E. Electonic Rapid Response: "Further Comments on Prof. Pocock's Paper" (with coworkers). *BMJ* (July 22, 2001).

35. Nassar, M. E. "Limitation of Benefit of CRT in Severe Failure." *BMJ* (May 30, 2003; February 10, 2004).

36. Nassar, M. E. Electronic Rapid Response: S. Goodacre, J. Nicholl, J., et al., "Randomized Controlled Trial and Economic Evaluation of a Chest Pain Unit Compared with Routine Care." *BMJ* 328 (2004): 254.

37. Nassar, M. E. Letter to the *ACP Observer*: "Performance Measures." *ACP-Observer* (March 2004).

38. Nassar, M. E. Electronic Rapid Response: "Another Clinical Perspective for the Evaluation of Chest Pain." *BMJ* (February 21, 2004).

39. Nassar, M. E. Electronic Rapid Response: James Heathcote, "Pancreatic Enzymes/Other Liver Function Tests in Reference to Clinical Review of Abnormal Liver Function after an Unplanned Consultation: Case Presentation," *BMJ* 329 (2004): 342.

40. Nassar, M. E. ACP/ Medical Knowledge Self-Assessment Test Program 13 Pre-Publication Test questions in *Neurology* answered (Spring 2004).

41. Nassar, M. E. ABIM-Cardiovascular Test 2004, 60 questions answered (June 16, 2004).

42. Nassar, M. E. Electronic Rapid Response: "Causes and Suggested Solution for Racial and Ethnic Disparities in Health Care 8/9/2004, in Reference to American College of Physicians": "Racial and Ethnic Disparities in Health Care: A Position Paper," *Ann Int Med* 141 (2004): 226–232.

43. Nassar, M. E. Commentary on "Rheumatic Heart Disease, Surgical Treatment of Mitral Stenosis" paper by John L. Wilson, MD; pathologic finding of a new auscultatory sign (2004). Work in progress; all rights reserved.

44. Nassar, M. E. "Racial and Ethnic Disparities in Health Care." *Ann Intern Med.* 142(2) (January 18, 2005): 153. Author reply 153-4.

45. Nassar, M. E. Electronic Rapid Response: "Clinical Approaches to Waist Circumference Reduction Requiring Further Study (as Treatment for Insulin Resistance in Type 2 DM)." *BMJ* (2005); 0:bmj.38429473310.AEv 1.

46. Nassar, M. E. "Reflections on the Life and Times of Professor Richard H. Scott, formerly Professor of Philosophy at the American University of Beirut." Read on his memorial celebration on May 7, 2005.

47. Nassar, M. E. Letter to Editor: "Comments on the 3rd and 4th Heart Sounds and Objective Data of Left Ventricular Dysfunction." *JAMA* 293 (2005): 2238–2244. Not published.

48. Nassar, M. E. Letter to Editor, *ACP Observer*, March 2004.

49. Young, J. Response to M. E. Nassar. Letter to Editor: *Today in Cardiology.* "Heart Failure" (May 2000).

50. Nassar, M. E. Electronic Rapid Response: "Lehman et al.: Cardiac Impairment or Heart Failure?" 331(7514) (2005): 415–416.

51. Nassar, M. E. Electronic Rapid Response: "Effects of Armed Conflict on Access to Emergency Health Care in Palestinian West Bank: Systematic Collection of Data in Emergency Departments." *BMJ* (October 26, 2006); 0: bmj 38793.695081.AEv1. A genuine paper by Dr. Rytter and colleagues.

52. Nassar, M. E. Electronic Rapid Response to Editor's Choice: "Fiona Godlee: Obviously" (October 18, 2006). "Physician Waiting before Action, Pending Evidence or Meta Analysis."

53. Nassar, M. E. Electronic Rapid Response to Editor: "Mozart's Death, a Diagnostic Dilemma." *Ann. Int. Med.* (August 24, 2009).

54. Nassar. M. E. "Hyposkillia: Deficiency of Clinical Skills." *Tex Heart Inst J.* 32(4) (2005): 623.

55. Nassar M. E. "Clinical evaluation of young athletes to prevent syncope or sudden death prior to exercise field events" Electronic rapid response to paper by Sofi and colleagues : cited in the BMJ 2008;337:a 346 and a second electronic response for the same BMJ cited paper " Why Exercise EKG

14 September 2008.

Index of Physicians and Their Contributions